Special Topics in Tropical Dermatology

Guest Editors

SCOTT A. NORTON, MD, MPH, MSc

AISHA SETHI, MD

DERMATOLOGIC CLINICS

www.derm.theclinics.com

Consulting Editor

BRUCE H. THIERS, MD

January 2011 • Volume 29 • Number 1

SAUNDERS an imprint of ELSEVIER, Inc.

W.B. SAUNDERS COMPANY
A Division of Elsevier Inc.

1600 John F. Kennedy Boulevard • Suite 1800 • Philadelphia, PA 19103-2899

http://www.theclinics.com

DERMATOLOGIC CLINICS Volume 29, Number 1
January 2011 ISSN 0733-8635, ISBN-13: 978-1-4557-0436-1

Editor: Carla Holloway
Developmental Editor: Jessica Demetriou

Dermatologic Clinics (ISSN 0733-8635) is published quarterly by Elsevier Inc., 360 Park Avenue South, New York, NY 10010-1710. Months of publication are January, April, July, and October. Business and editorial offices: 1600 John F. Kennedy Blvd., Suite 1800, Philadelphia, PA 19103-2899. Customer service office: 11830 Westline Drive, St. Louis, MO 63146. Periodicals postage paid at New York, NY, and additional mailing offices. Subscription prices are USD 317.00 per year for US individuals, USD 474.00 per year for US institutions, USD 371.00 per year for Canadian individuals, USD 568.00 per year for Canadian institutions, USD 434.00 per year for international individuals, USD 568.00 per year for international institutions, USD 148.00 per year for US students/residents, and USD 214.00 per year for Canadian and international students/residents. International air speed delivery is included in all *Clinics* subscription prices. All prices are subject to change without notice. **POSTMASTER:** Send address changes to *Dermatologic Clinics*, Elsevier Health Sciences Division, Subscription Customer Service, 3251 Riverport Lane, Maryland Heights, MO 63043. **Customer Service: 1-800-654-2452 (U.S. and Canada); 314-447-8871 (outside U.S. and Canada). Fax: 314-447-8029.** E-mail: journalscustomerservice-usa@elsevier.com (for print support); journalsonlinesupport-usa@elsevier.com (for online support).

Reprints. For copies of 100 or more, of articles in this publication, please contact the Commercial Reprints Department, Elsevier Inc., 360 Park Avenue South, New York, New York 10010-1710. Tel.: (212) 633-3813; Fax: (212) 462-1935; Email: repritns@elsevier.com.

The *Dermatologic Clinics* is covered in *MEDLINE/PubMed (Index Medicus)*, *Current Contents/Clinical Medicine*, *Excerpta Medica*, *Chemical Abstracts*, and *ISI/BIOMED*.

Printed and bound by CPI Group (UK) Ltd, Croydon, CR0 4YY

Transferred to Digital Print 2011

Contributors

CONSULTING EDITOR

BRUCE H. THIERS, MD
Professor and Chairman, Department
of Dermatology and Dermatologic Surgery,
Medical University of South Carolina,
Charleston, South Carolina

GUEST EDITORS

AISHA SETHI, MD
Assistant Professor of Medicine, Associate
Residency Program Director, University
of Chicago, Section of Dermatology,
Chicago, Illinois

SCOTT A. NORTON, MD, MPH, MSc
Division of Dermatology, Department of Medicine,
Georgetown University Hospital, Washington, DC;
Clinical Consultant, Dermatology Branch, National
Cancer Institute, National Institutes of Health,
Bethesda, Maryland; Consultant in Dermatology
and Tropical Medicine, Peace Corps,
Washington, DC

AUTHORS

HABIBUL AHSAN, MD, MMedSc
Professor, Departments of Medicine and Human
Genetics and Cancer Research Center, University
of Chicago, Chicago, Illinois

ERIN HUIRAS AMERSON, MD
Department of Dermatology, University
of California, San Francisco, San Francisco,
California

DAVID ANSDELL, BA
John A. Burns School of Medicine, University
of Hawaii, Honolulu, Hawaii

JACK L. ARBISER, MD, PhD
Professor, Department of Dermatology,
Emory University School of Medicine, Atlanta;
Chief of Service, Division of Dermatology,
Atlanta Veterans Administration Medical Center,
Decatur, Georgia

RICARDO L. BERRIOS, MD
Post-Doctoral Fellow, Department of
Dermatology, Emory University School
of Medicine, Atlanta, Georgia

RON BIRNBAUM, MD
Chief Resident in Dermatology, Los Angeles
Biomedical Research Institute at Harbor-UCLA
Medical Center, Torrance, California

**JONATHAN R. CARAPETIS, MBBS, FRACP,
PhD, MPH**
Pediatric Infectious Diseases Physician, Royal
Darwin Hospital; Director, Child Health, Menzies
School of Health Research, Casuarina, Darwin,
Northern Territory, Australia

NOAH CRAFT, MD, PhD, DTM&H
Assistant Professor of Dermatology and Infectious
Disease, Los Angeles Biomedical Research
Institute at Harbor-UCLA Medical Center,
Torrance; David Geffen School of Medicine at the
University of California, Los Angeles,
Los Angeles, California

ANDRES E. CRUZ-INIGO, MD
Scripps Mercy Hospital, San Diego, California

AMISH J. DAVE, MD
Resident, Department of Medicine, Stanford
University School of Medicine, Stanford, California

SEYDOU DOUMBIA, MD, PhD
Malaria Research Training Center, University
of Bamako, Bamako, Mali

**KENNETH GALECKAS, MD, FAAD, LCDR,
MC, USN**
Staff Dermatologist, Department of Dermatology,
National Naval Medical Center; Assistant
Professor of Dermatology, Uniformed Services
University of the Health Sciences, Bethesda,
Maryland

CAMILLE E. INTROCASO, MD
Department of Dermatology, Pennsylvania
Hospital; Pennsylvania Center for Dermatology,
Philadelphia, Pennsylvania

ADAM W. JENNEY, MBBS, FRACP, PhD
Epidemiologist, Centre for International Child
Health, University of Melbourne; Infectious
Diseases Physician, Infectious Diseases Unit,
The Alfred Hospital, Melbourne, Victoria,
Australia

SOMITA KEITA, MD
Centre National d'Appui a la lutte contre la
Maladie (CNAM), Bamako, Mali

CARRIE L. KOVARIK, MD
Assistant Professor of Dermatology and
Infectious Disease, Department of Dermatology;
Division of Infectious Disease, Department
of Internal Medicine, Hospital of the University
of Pennsylvania, Philadelphia, Pennsylvania

ROOPAL V. KUNDU, MD
Department of Dermatology, Northwestern
University Feinberg School of Medicine,
Chicago, Illinois

BARRY LADIZINSKI, MD
Department of Internal Medicine, Yale University
School of Medicine, New Haven, Connecticut

SABA M. LAMBERT, MBBS
London School of Hygiene and Tropical Medicine,
London, United Kingdom

JOSEPH V. LILLIS, MD
Assistant Professor, Division of Dermatology,
Department of Medicine, University of
California, San Diego Medical Center,
San Diego, California

DIANA N.J. LOCKWOOD, MD, FRCP
London School of Hygiene and Tropical Medicine,
London, United Kingdom

OMAR LUPI, MD, PhD
Dermatology Department, Federal University
of the State of Rio de Janeiro (UNI-RIO);
Chairman, Dermatology Department,
Policlínica Geral do Rio de Janeiro;
Immunology Department, Federal University
of Rio de Janeiro (UFRJ), Rio de Janeiro, Brazil

TOBY A. MAURER, MD
Department of Dermatology, University
of California, San Francisco, San Francisco,
California

WAYNE M. MEYERS, MD, PhD
Department of Environmental and Infectious
Disease Sciences, Armed Forces Institute
of Pathology, Washington, DC

NISHA MISTRY, MD
Department of Dermatology and Skin Science,
University of British Columbia, Vancouver,
British Columbia, Canada

ALDO MORRONE, MD, PhD
Director General, National Institute for Health,
Migration and Poverty, Roma, Italy

EVA RAWLINGS PARKER, MD
Franklin Dermatology Group, Franklin, Tennessee

CARLOS PAZ, MD, PhD
Section of Dermatology, University of Chicago,
Chicago, Illinois

FRANÇOISE PORTAELS, PhD
Professor, Mycobacteriology Unit, Department
of Microbiology, Institute of Tropical Medicine,
Antwerp, Belgium

ARLENE M. RUIZ DE LUZURIAGA, MD, MPH
Clinical Associate of Medicine, Section
of Dermatology, Department of Medicine,
University of Chicago Medical Center,
Chicago, Illinois

AISHA SETHI, MD
Assistant Professor of Medicine, Associate
Residency Program Director, University of
Chicago, Section of Dermatology, Chicago,
Illinois

CHRISTOPHER R. SHEA, MD
Professor and Chief, Section of Dermatology, Department of Medicine, University of Chicago Medical Center, Chicago, Illinois

ANDREW C. STEER, MBBS, FRACP, PhD
Senior Research Fellow, Centre for International Health, University of Melbourne; Pediatric Infectious Diseases Physician, Department of Paediatrics, Centre for International Child Health, Royal Children's Hospital, Melbourne, Victoria, Australia

STEVEN Y.C. TONG, MBBS, FRACP, PhD
Senior Research Fellow, Tropical and Emerging Infectious Diseases, Menzies School of Health Research, Casuarina, Darwin; Infectious Diseases Physician, Infectious Diseases Department, Royal Darwin Hospital, Tiwi, Northern Territory, Australia

DOUGLAS S. WALSH, MD
Department of Immunology and Medicine, United States Army Medical Component, Armed Forces Research Institute of Medical Sciences (AFRIMS), Bangkok, Thailand

Contents

> Buruli ulcer (BU), caused by the environmental organism *Mycobacterium ulcerans* and characterized by necrotizing skin and bone lesions, poses important public health issues as the third most common mycobacterial infection in humans. Pathogenesis of *M ulcerans* is mediated by mycolactone, a necrotizing immunosuppressive toxin. First-line therapy for BU is rifampin plus streptomycin, sometimes with surgery. New insights into the pathogenesis of BU should improve control strategies.

> Approximately 10% of the island population of Satowan (population, 650 persons), a small, remote coral island in the central Pacific, suffers from an acquired, chronic, disfiguring skin condition known locally as "spam." This skin disease has affected the island population since shortly after World War II. An investigation in 2007 revealed that this skin disease is caused by a nontuberculous mycobacterial infection closely related to *Mycobacterium marinum*. This article reviews the fascinating history of this skin disease on Satowan, its distinctive clinical presentation, and recommendations for diagnosis and treatment of clinically similar skin lesions in Pacific Islanders.

> On the 12th of January 2010, Haiti was struck by a 7.0 Richter magnitude earthquake that devastated its already fragile capital region. Approximately 230,000 people died immediately or during ensuing weeks, mostly due to acute trauma. Countless others suffered significant life- or limb-threatening injuries. As a part of the United States' response to this tragedy, eventually named Operation Unified Response, the United States Navy deployed hundreds of physicians and other medical response individuals on a hospital ship. Operation Unified Response was a military joint task force operation augmented by governmental and nongovernmental organizations. Its mission was to bring medical and logistical support to the region.

> Skin and soft tissue infections (SSTI) caused by *Staphylococcus aureus* are very common, particularly in children, in tropical regions. The proportion of *S aureus* SSTI caused by community-associated methicillin-resistant *S aureus* (CA-MRSA) varies according to region, but is up to 25% in some areas. There are diverse

CA-MRSA clones, including several that harbor Panton-Valentine leukocidin. Key predisposing factors for staphylococcal infections are scabies infestation, overcrowding, poor hygiene, and inadequate water supplies. In the setting of a community outbreak of staphylococcal SSTI, interventions intended to improve personal and community hygiene are likely to be the most practical, effective, and achievable. Options for oral treatment of clinical infections caused by CA-MRSA include clindamycin and trimethoprim-sulfamethoxazole. Although rapid diagnostics are now available, and 2 vaccines have reached clinical trials, neither of these is likely to be of use in tropical, developing regions in the near future.

Arboviruses continue to be a significant source of disease, especially in regions where their insect hosts are endemic. This article highlights these diseases, with particular focus on dengue, yellow fever, and viral hemorrhagic fever. A general background is provided, as well information concerning diagnosis and treatment.

The human immunodeficiency virus (HIV) pandemic has disproportionately affected tropical regions of the world, where dermatoses, such as leprosy and leishmaniasis, rarely encountered in temperate climates, are endemic. Although the introduction of highly active antiretroviral therapy (HAART) has been lifesaving, a few patients undergoing HAART experience clinical deterioration caused by immune reconstitution inflammatory syndrome (IRIS). This article explores the range of tropical dermatoses that are reported to date with associated IRIS events.

Arsenic is considered a Class I human carcinogen by the International Agency for Research on Cancer because of its increased risk for skin cancer, as well as internal cancers, such as lung and bladder cancer. Arsenic contamination of drinking water in Bangladesh has been called the "largest mass poisoning of a population in history." This inorganic arsenic contamination is of natural origin, with arsenic thought to be released to the groundwater from the surrounding sediment. Arsenicosis and its risk factors and prevention and management are discussed in this article.

Chagas disease, or American trypanosomiasis, is a parasitic infection caused by the flagellate protozoan *Trypanosoma cruzi*, an organism that is endemic to Latin America. While Chagas disease is primarily a vector-borne illness, new cases are emerging in non-endemic areas due to globalization of immigration and non-vectorial transmission routes. This article discusses the mode of transmission, evolving epidemiology, pathogenesis, diagnosis, treatment and prevention and control of the disease.

Camille E. Introcaso and Carrie L. Kovarik

In 2008, the American Academy of Dermatology began sponsoring North American dermatology residents to travel to Botswana in sub-Saharan Africa and spend 4 to 6 weeks working with the Botswana-UPenn Partnership, the Baylor International Pediatrics AIDS Initiative, Princess Marina Hospital, and surrounding smaller district hospitals. During their time in Botswana, the residents staff the busy outpatient dermatology clinic and see adult and pediatric inpatients at Princess Marina Hospital in Gaborone, the capital city. The residents also travel to 4 rural hospitals to provide clinical services to patient and education to local health care providers. The program goals include providing direct care to the people of Botswana, capacity-building through dermatologic education for local clinicians, and educating the residents about delivering dermatologic care in resource-limited and culturally diverse settings and using teledermatology consulting services. Since the start of the program, more than 1500 patients have been seen, and 35 residents would have completed the program by the end of 2010.

Ricardo L. Berrios and Jack L. Arbiser

The term pyoderma encompasses a variety of distinct entities including impetigo (bullous and nonbullous), erysipelas, cellulitis, folliculitis, and staphylococcal scalded skin syndrome. Treatment of pyodermas centers around wound care and appropriate antibiotic selection. Triphenylmethane dyes, such as gentian violet, represent a unique group of compounds that act as antiseptics and have shown clinical efficacy as antibiotics in a variety of pyodermas, including those secondary to methicillin-resistant *Staphylococcus aureus*. Given their low cost, ease of application, and favorable side effect profile, triphenylmethanes must be considered legitimate treatment options for pyodermas, particularly in the face of continued and emerging bacterial resistance.

Carlos Paz, Seydou Doumbia, Somita Keita, and Aisha Sethi

While not as common as in other parts of the world, cutaneous leishmaniasis is endemic to countries in Africa, particularly in the north, central, east, and south. Sporadic case reports of cutaneous leishmaniasis in countries spanning West Africa have allowed scientists to propose an endemic belt in sub-Saharan Africa ranging from Senegal to Cameroon. While the presence of cutaneous leishmaniasis in West Africa is well established, there is a paucity of data regarding the parasite species, vector, and reservoir responsible for the disease in this part of the continent. This article focuses on cutaneous leishmaniasis in Mali, West Africa.

Andres E. Cruz-Inigo, Barry Ladizinski, and Aisha Sethi

Oculocutaneous albinism is an autosomal recessive disorder characterized by a lack of pigment in the hair, skin, and eyes. Albinism is caused by defective or absent tyrosinase, an enzyme necessary for melanogenesis. Although rare in the western world, albinism is quite common in sub-Saharan Africa, likely as a result of consanguinity. Albinism has long been associated with stigma and superstitions, such as the belief that a white man impregnated the mother or that the child is the ghost of a European colonist. Recently, a notion has emerged that albino body parts are good-luck charms or possess magical powers. These body parts may be sold for as much as $75,000 on the black market. As a result there have been over 100 albino murders in Tanzania, Burundi, and other parts of Africa in the past decade, which is now beginning to garner international attention and thus prompting novel legislation. To ameliorate the plight of individuals with albinism in Africa, a coordinated effort must be organized, involving medical professionals (dermatologists, ophthalmologists, oncologists), public health advocates and educators, social workers, human rights and antidiscrimination activists, law-enforcement agencies, and governmental support groups. The main issues that should be addressed include skin cancer prevention education, stigma and discrimination denouncement, and swift prosecution of albino hunters and their sponsors.

Despite the ubiquity and severity of parasitic diseases and our desire to prevent them, there are no effective antiparasitic vaccines in widespread clinical use. This review focuses on strategies for development of a vaccine against cutaneous leishmaniasis as a representative parasitic disease of paramount interest to dermatologists and all who care for patients who live in or travel to the developing world. Any effective strategy will require attention to the central role that host innate immunity plays during induction of durable resistance to these virulent protozoa. The cell types, receptors, and molecules of the innate immune system that will likely play a role in any effective vaccine against cutaneous leishmaniasis are reviewed.

Female genital mutilation (FGM) has become more common in the United States with increased immigration to the United States of individuals from areas where the practice is endemic. Although the root causes of FGM may be multiple, the practice is banned in the United States on all women under age 18 and is increasingly being outlawed by individual state legislatures. American dermatologists should expect to see a growing number of patients having undergone FGM who may present with complications ranging from keloids and epidermal cysts to clitoral neuromas and abscess formation. While treatment of such complications is often elusive and unsuccessful, recognition of the practice may prevent future patient abuse and death. The eradication of FGM will require the concerted efforts of many individuals, both within and outside of the health care field, with dermatologists poised to play a crucial role in diagnosis and management in the near future.

Hyperpigmentation disorders and skin lightening treatments have a significant impact on the dermatologic, physiologic, psychologic, economic, social, and cultural aspects of life. Skin lightening compounds, such as hydroquinone and topical corticosteroids, are often used to treat hyperpigmentation disorders, such as melasma, or lighten skin for cosmetic purposes. Despite their established effectiveness, a multitude of dermatologic and systemic complications have been associated with these agents. Regulatory agencies have also recognized the adverse effects of skin lighteners and many countries around the world now forbid the production and sale of these compounds, although this prohibition has not significantly curtailed distribution. Dermatologists and users of cosmetic products should be aware of the various components in bleaching compounds, their potential adverse effects, and alternative options for skin lightening.

Coinfection with human immunodeficiency virus (HIV) has a major effect on the natural history of many infectious diseases, particularly mycobacterial diseases. Early in the HIV epidemic, it was predicted that HIV infection would worsen leprosy outcomes, with more patients developing lepromatous disease, an impaired response to multidrug therapy and fewer reactions. However, studies on the epidemiologic and clinical aspects of leprosy suggest that the course of leprosy in coinfected patients has not been greatly altered by HIV. In contrast, initiation of antiretroviral treatment has been reported to be associated with activation of subclinical *Mycobacterium leprae* infection and exacerbation of existing leprosy lesions. With regular new discoveries about the interaction of leprosy and HIV, the need to maintain research in this field is of considerable importance.

Dermatologic Clinics

THE CLINICS ARE NOW AVAILABLE ONLINE!

Access your subscription at:
www.theclinics.com

Preface
Special Topics in Tropical Dermatology

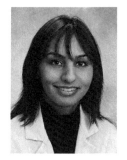

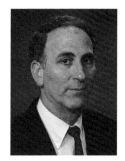

Aisha Sethi, MD   Scott A. Norton, MD, MPH, MSc
Guest Editors

Thank you for pausing to read this introduction. This is not your typical publication on *Tropical Dermatology*. This is something new.

We expect that every reader will find several topics in this issue to be entirely new to them—and we believe that readers will find the topics fascinating, the content instructive, and the prose clear.

Typically, journal articles on tropical dermatology provide a general overview of specific cutaneous infectious diseases. We won't do that here; this issue is devoted to 16 focused topics, including many cultural practices and noninfectious dermatologic conditions that challenge the health of individuals and the social fabric of communities in tropical regions.

Some of the most important assaults on health in the developing world are the direct result of long-ingrained cultural practices and human behaviors. For example, female genital mutilation (the intentional alteration of a young woman's external genitalia), practiced in societies across much of Africa and parts of Asia, has huge medical, societal, and reproductive consequences. Another example takes place in parts of East Africa where albinism is relatively common. In tropical agrarian societies, albinos suffer from intense sun exposure and the resultant, often lethal, skin cancers. They also suffer from prejudice and superstition in school, work, and marriage—and here we read that they are targets of a horrific, murderous trade in body parts, which are valued for their putative metaphysical properties.

Irrespective of the underlying motivations, in many parts of the world, people with medium or dark complexions attempt to lighten their skin, often using compounds that are pharmacologically dangerous or, simply put, pure toxins. In this volume, we read about these and more topics on the boundary of skin and society.

There is more to understanding these conditions than simply studying anatomic modifications and pigment pharmacology. There are complex societal issues surrounding these cultural practices, the treatment of their detrimental consequences, and, preferably, their prevention.

There are steady advances in our understanding of specific tropical infectious diseases and we present the newest material for several conditions, including two, Buruli ulcer and Chagas disease, that the World Health Organization has identified as serious emerging infections. Because of population shifts and global environmental variation, these infectious diseases have greatly expanded their natural endemic borders.

Progress in treating tropical disorders requires the development of newer and better medical therapies. One such example is the single-dose strategy to treat leprosy. Is it possible that a day's worth of medication—a few, widely available tablets—will revolutionize the treatment of leprosy on a par with the therapeutic changes

Dermatol Clin 29 (2011) xiii–xiv
doi:10.1016/j.det.2010.10.001

brought about by the invention of sulfone compounds, such as dapsone? Along a different line, the increasingly widespread use of highly active antiretroviral therapies in the developing world has created the unintended challenge of immune reconstitution inflammatory syndrome, which frequently appears as one's immune system regains its ability to fight latent or quiescent infections. Not all pharmacologic advances require new therapies, however. For example, gentian violet, a topical aniline dye used for more than a century as a first-line topical anti-infective throughout the developing world, might just be the right stuff for treating those ubiquitous and inevitable tropical pyodermas.

Other articles tell us about the cutaneous effects of environmental hazards and natural disasters, such as the high levels of arsenic in Bangladesh's drinking water and the 2010 Haiti earthquake, respectively. Here, too, we learn about the duties of a US Navy dermatologist assigned to a hospital ship off Port-au-Prince. Two additional articles describe ways that dermatologists from developed nations can bring their skills to regions in need of cutaneous medicine. The American Academy of Dermatology participates in a program that permits one resident per month to serve as the dermatologist at the national children's hospital in Botswana. We learn also about the investigation to uncover the identity of the pathogen causing a strange skin infection on one of the world's smallest and most remote islands.

The authors whom we assembled to prepare these articles are among the world's experts, including the authorities to whom the World Health Organization turns with its questions about these conditions. We wish to thank our contributors for their splendid submissions and the readers for taking time to read these special topics in tropical dermatology.

Aisha Sethi, MD
Section of Dermatology
University of Chicago
5841 South Maryland Avenue, MC 5067
Chicago, IL 60637, USA

Scott A. Norton, MD, MPH, MSc
Dermatology Division
Georgetown University Hospital
3800 Reservoir Road, NW
Washington, DC 20007, USA

E-mail addresses:
asethi@medicine.bsd.uchicago.edu (A. Sethi)
scottanorton@gmail.com (S.A. Norton)

Buruli Ulcer: Advances in Understanding *Mycobacterium ulcerans* Infection

Douglas S. Walsh, MD[a],*, Françoise Portaels, PhD[b],
Wayne M. Meyers, MD, PhD[c]

KEYWORDS

- Buruli ulcer • *Mycobacterium ulcerans* • Emerging disease
- Skin disease • Mycolactone

Buruli ulcer (BU), the third most common mycobacterial infection in humans next to tuberculosis and leprosy, is an emerging infection caused by *Mycobacterium ulcerans*. BU is characterized by indolent, typically painless necrotizing skin lesions (**Figs. 1** and **2**A). Approximately 10% of patients develop bone involvement subjacent to skin lesions or metastatic osteomyelitis from lymphohematogenous spread of *M ulcerans* (see **Fig. 2**B). Pathogenesis is mediated by mycolactone, a diffusible, necrotizing, immunosuppressive, polyketide-derived macrolide toxin secreted by *M ulcerans*.[1] In 1962, the disease was named after Buruli County, Uganda, now called Nakasongola District, where the epidemic was documented first. Other names include Bairnsdale, Kakerifu, Kasongo, or Searls' ulcer.

EPIDEMIOLOGY

In 1998, the World Health Organization (WHO) recognized BU as a reemerging infectious disease in West and Central Africa, with a significant public health impact.[2] The reported incidence rates of BU are highest in West Africa, especially Benin, Ghana, and Côte d'Ivoire. However, BU is reported in about 30 countries (**Fig. 3**), and growing evidence suggests that BU is more widespread than earlier thought.[3] BU prevails in rural tropical wetlands, especially areas with stagnant water, including ponds and swamps. However, BU is also acquired without wetland exposure.

The rapid reemergence of BU, beginning in the early 1980s, particularly in areas where people are engaged in manual agriculture in wetlands, may be attributable to the man-made alterations to the environment, such as deforestation and other topographic alterations, which increase the amount of wetlands. Changes in global temperature and precipitation patterns further promote the reemergence of BU.

The WHO reports indicate that more than 5000 people are diagnosed with BU annually, but many cases are undiagnosed because of the geopolitical and socioeconomic factors in endemic countries. Children (5–15 years old) have the highest incidence of BU, with most lesions on the lower extremities. BU is a growing

Disclosure: The authors have nothing to disclose.

Disclaimer: The views expressed in this article are those of the author (D.S.W.) and do not reflect the official policy of the Department of the Army, Department of Defense, or the US government.

[a] Department of Immunology and Medicine, United States Army Medical Component, Armed Forces Research Institute of Medical Sciences (AFRIMS), 315/6 Rajvithi Road, Bangkok 10400, Thailand

[b] Mycobacteriology Unit, Department of Microbiology, Institute of Tropical Medicine, Nationalestraat 155, B-2000 Antwerp, Belgium

[c] Department of Environmental and Infectious Disease Sciences, Armed Forces Institute of Pathology, Washington, DC 20306, USA

* Corresponding author.

E-mail address: douglas.walsh@afrims.org

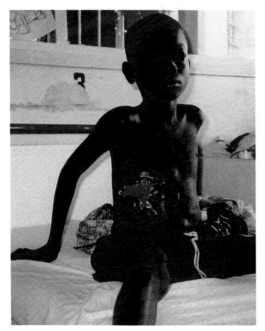

Fig. 1. Plaque of BU on the right flank of a Ghanaian boy. The lesion has characteristic rolled borders and is remarkably stellate, a feature of some plaques.

public health problem, with psychosocial and socioeconomic implications in endemic regions. Up to 60% of patients with BU suffer from disabling and stigmatizing sequelae, including scarring, contractures, and bone destruction.[4] Minimizing disability through treatment, both antimicrobial and surgical, and physiotherapy is, therefore, important in BU management. Imported BU is occasionally diagnosed in the United States, Canada, and Europe.[5]

BU is directly related to environmental factors and thus considered noncontagious.[6] The most possible mode of transmission is local, minor, often unnoticed skin trauma that permits inoculation of *M ulcerans*. The estimated incubation period is 2 to 3 months. Because *M ulcerans* DNA is detectable in some aquatic insects, the role of insects as vectors that infect humans by biting is under investigation.[7] In Australia, some investigators propose that BU is a zoonosis transmitted by mosquitoes from indigenous marsupials (eg, possums and koalas) to humans. *M ulcerans* DNA was found in mosquitoes during an outbreak of BU in humans in Australia, and the seasonal incidence of BU in humans correlates with that of notifiable arthropod-borne diseases in Victoria.[8] In Africa, terrestrial mammals are being investigated as reservoirs of *M ulcerans*.[9]

Risk factors for BU within endemic areas include failure to wear protective clothing, exposure to unprotected natural water sources, and inadequate care of minor skin wounds.[10,11] Human immunodeficiency virus seropositivity may increase the risk for BU or be associated with aggressive BU.[12]

BCG vaccination has some effect on BU. Several reports suggest that BCG vaccination provides some protection against BU, for 6 to 12 months after vaccination, and that neonatal BCG vaccination reduces the risk of BU osteomyelitis in those who acquire BU as children or adults.[13–15] However, a case-control study concluded that BCG vaccination is not protective against BU.[16] Prophylactic and therapeutic vaccines based on DNA engineering and virulence factors, including mycolactone, are under study (BuruliVac Project).[17] Intravenous immunoglobulin to neutralize mycolactone is not available.

MICROBIOLOGY OF *M ULCERANS*

Standard and real-time polymerase chain reaction (PCR) techniques have been used to identify *M ulcerans*, primarily by detecting 2 *M ulcerans* insertion sequences (IS*2404* and IS*2606*), in the environment in Australia and West Africa.[18] Improved *M ulcerans* DNA extraction procedures enhance environmental

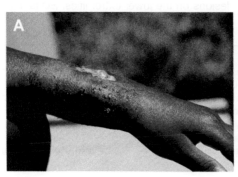
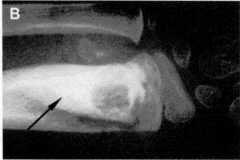

Fig. 2. (*A*) Plaque of BU on the forearm of a Congolese boy invaded the deep tissues and bone, causing contiguous osteomyelitis. (*B*) Radiograph shows contiguous reactive osteitis and necrosis of the cortex of the radius, with formation of a large sequestrum (*arrow*).

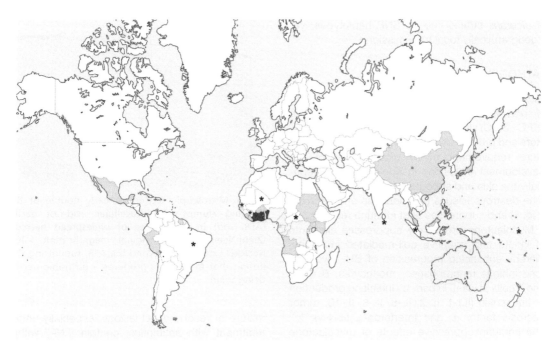

Fig. 3. Distribution of BU by country, as of 2010. Relative endemicity is denoted as high (*red*), moderate (*yellow*), and low (*green*); asterisks denote countries with suspected cases. Imported BU is occasionally diagnosed in the United States, Canada, and Europe.

detection, thereby advancing the understanding of reservoirs.[19] Portaels and colleagues[20] reported the first direct isolation of *M ulcerans* from nature in 2008 from a water strider, an aquatic insect that does not bite humans.

Unlike *M leprae* and *M tuberculosis* (the pathogens for leprosy and tuberculosis, respectively), *M ulcerans* produces a necrotizing, immunosuppressive, polyketide-derived macrolide toxin, called mycolactone.[1] Genes in a virulence plasmid of *M ulcerans*, controlled by SigA-like promoters,[21] encode for the synthesis of mycolactone. Identification of SigA-like promoters led to the development of *M ulcerans*–green fluorescent protein. This tagged protein linking fluorescence with toxin gene expression is a potential tool for studying BU pathogenesis and transmission.[21]

M ulcerans shares some environmental, molecular, and clinical features with *M marinum*, a water-associated organism that causes granulomatous skin lesions in humans, often called "swimming pool" or "fish tank" granuloma. Comparative genomics indicate that *M ulcerans* likely diverged from *M marinum*, acquiring a 174-kb virulence plasmid (pMUM001) with genes coding for mycolactone production and 10 proteins, all potential targets for vaccine development or serodiagnosis.[22] Accordingly, phenolic mycosides of *M ulcerans* and *M marinum* are

identical, and sequences for the 16S ribosomal RNA (rRNA) gene are nearly identical.[6] As *M ulcerans* evolved toward becoming an intracellular organism, like *M marinum*, nonessential genes were lost, which may have increased the pathogenicity.[22]

Gene sequences of the 3′ end of the 16S rRNA of *M ulcerans* vary by geographic origin, dividing *M ulcerans* broadly into African, American, Asian, and Australian strains, with many substrains on each continent.[23] Each major strain generally differs in clinical presentation, mycolactone type and virulence, and host immune responses.[24] Mycolactone type coding by geographic origin includes A/B (Africa, the most pathogenic), C (Asia, Australia), and D (Asia).[1]

Molecular genetic techniques are slowly unraveling the evolution of *M ulcerans*. *M ulcerans* isolates from localized foci within endemic regions often show a high degree of genomic similarity (ie, clonal populations) with a lack of insertional-deletional genomic polymorphisms, underscoring a requirement for single-nucleotide polymorphism (SNP) analysis to differentiate substrains of *M ulcerans* within those areas.[25] Identifying SNPs and establishing SNP typing assays are increasingly defining the microepidemiology, genetic diversity, and evolution of *M ulcerans*.[26,27] For example, SNP analyses of *M ulcerans* in Ghana differentiate 54

M ulcerans strains into 13 SNP haplotypes, yet a geographically focal transmission.[27,28]

PATHOGENESIS AND IMMUNITY

Initial infection is primarily related to 2 properties of *M ulcerans*: optimal growth at temperatures (30°C–33°C) slightly below the core body temperature and production of mycolactone. The temperature requirement of *M ulcerans* favors the development of lesions in cooler tissues, especially the skin and subcutaneous tissue. Mycolactone destroys tissues by apoptosis and necrosis (**Fig. 4**) and suppresses host immune responses.[1]

Mycolactone profoundly suppresses elements of innate and adaptive cell-mediated immunity, thereby enhancing progression of BU. Mycolactone inhibits macrophages, monocytes, B cells, and T cells at least, in part, by inhibiting production of interleukin (IL)-1, IL-2, IL-6, IL-8, IL-10, tumor necrosis factor α, and interferon-γ (IFN-γ).[29,30] The immunosuppressive effects of mycolactone extend beyond skin lesions to circulating leukocytes and lymphoid organs.[31] Peripheral whole-blood samples from patients with active BU, when stimulated with mitogens, produce comparatively smaller amounts of helper T cell (T_H) 1, T_H2, and T_H17 cytokines.[32]

The clinical and histopathologic features of BU suggest an immunologic spectrum of host responses over time, which may be relevant for vaccine strategies. Early progressive ulcers generate abundant IL-10 with little inflammation (T_H2 response) and numerous, often extracellular, *M ulcerans* (**Fig. 5**) within areas of coagulation necrosis. Necrosis reflects mycolactone-induced death of tissue and inflammatory cells. In contrast,

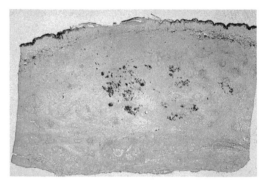

Fig. 5. Microscopic section of early nodule of BU showing clumps of extracellular acid-fast bacilli (AFB, *red*) in the center of widespread necrosis (Ziehl-Neelsen stain, original magnification ×40). Necrosis extends far beyond the AFB, supporting the notion that *M ulcerans* produces a diffusible necrotizing toxin.

mature or resolving BU lesions, especially under treatment with antibiotics, contain IFN-γ within granulomatous inflammation, organizing lymphoid aggregates, and typically intracellular *M ulcerans*, consistent with a T_H1, delayed-type hypersensitivity (DTH) response.[1,33,34] DTH in these patients, but not those with early BU or uninfected persons, is verified by skin test reactivity against burulin, a sonicate of *M ulcerans*.[35] Minor BU may self-heal early, suggesting elements of high host resistance.

CLINICAL FEATURES AND DIAGNOSIS

BU presents as a spectrum of localized or disseminated clinical forms, with variable natural history (**Fig. 6**). Early lesions are usually papular, nodular, or edematous, progressing to ulcers with rolled borders, spreading laterally. Most ulcers are painless unless secondarily infected. Fever and lymphadenopathy are rare. Experienced workers may

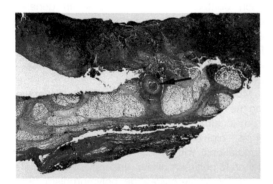

Fig. 4. Microscopic section of the undermined edge of a major BU. Note contiguous coagulation necrosis of the panniculus and fascia and vasculitis with thrombosis of a medium-sized vessel (*arrow*) (hematoxylin-eosin, original magnification ×40). A mild host inflammatory response is consistent with a toxin-mediated process.

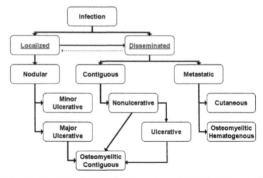

Fig. 6. Proposed classification and natural history of untreated clinical forms of active BU.

correctly diagnose some BU lesions on clinical features alone, but there is often discord between clinical impression and laboratory results because of incorrect clinical diagnosis, inadequate sampling, or laboratory errors. Important entities in the differential diagnosis of ulcerative and edematous BU include tropical phagedenic ulcer and necrotizing fasciitis, respectively.[36] Both these conditions, unlike BU, are painful. Many other conditions resemble BU, underscoring the importance of laboratory confirmation. Radiographic examination is indicated when bone involvement is suspected.

The 4 diagnostic laboratory tests for BU are (1) direct smear (with acid-fast stains auramine O or Ziehl-Neelsen), (2) culture, (3) histopathology, and (4) PCR. Estimated sensitivities for these techniques range from 60% or lesser to more than 90%. PCR, currently available only in research laboratories, is considered the most reliable method for all lesion subtypes,[37] followed by histopathology, culture, and direct smear. Lesion sampling techniques include swabbing, punch biopsy, and, as a less-invasive alternative to biopsy, fine-needle aspiration (FNA). PCR is highly sensitive when applied to swabbed material from ulcers and to biopsies and FNAs of nonulcerative lesions.[38] The targets of PCR, IS*2404* and IS*2606*, may be present in other pathogenic mycobacteria, such as *M marinum*; so clinical features or variable number of tandem repeat assays may discriminate *M ulcerans* from other species.[39]

Among the non-PCR diagnostic methods, histopathology is useful to confirm BU or generate a differential diagnosis when unconfirmed. Culture is recommended for tracking treatment response, often a concern in clinical trials.[38] Pharmacologic assays to detect mycolactone in the tissues infected with *M ulcerans* may become a diagnostic adjunct to culture.[40] Direct smears are useful at the community level. Rapid diagnostic tests for use in the field, to detect mycolactone or *M ulcerans*–specific proteins in lesional or other biologic fluids, are in early development.

Regardless of the test or sampling method, at least 2 sites per lesion suspicious for BU should be sampled; this process increases sensitivity over a single sample by up to 25%. When confronted with possible new geographic foci of BU, confirmation by PCR and at least 1 of the other 3 tests is advised.

TREATMENT

Historically, treatment of BU has been surgical excision of the affected tissues, correction of wound defects, and, if available, rehabilitative physiotherapy. Bone and joint lesions are given priority. By the 1970s, rifampin was known to heal most small BU lesions. However, until 2005, antibiotics remained a largely perioperative adjunctive therapy, aimed at reducing dissemination and recurrence or minimizing tissue excision.[41] The role of adjunctive antibiotic therapy for BU that is otherwise surgically excised remains unclear.[42] Other treatment methods, such as local heat, explored decades ago, may become practical as application systems are simplified.[43]

In 2004, with increasing BU incidence and limited surgical resources in Africa, supported by experimental and encouraging preliminary human data,[44] the WHO advocated a provisional antibiotic regimen for BU, comprising oral rifampin (10 mg/kg) plus intramuscular streptomycin (15 mg/kg), both given daily for 8 weeks under supervision.[45] Amikacin (15 mg/kg) can be substituted for streptomycin, administered intramuscularly or intravenously. Important contraindications and side effects for these drugs are described elsewhere.[45] As general guidelines, patients with lesions less than 5 cm in diameter (category I, small) receive antibiotics alone and those with lesions 5 to 15 cm in diameter (category II, moderate) receive 4 weeks of antibiotics and then undergo surgery, if necessary, followed by 4 more weeks of antibiotics. Patients with lesions more than 15 cm in diameter (category III, advanced) are treated with antibiotics for at least 1 week before surgery; the antibiotics are then continued for a total of 8 weeks. Follow-up of all patients is advised for an additional 10 months to assess for cure and complications.

Case series studies of rifampin plus streptomycin for small and moderate BU conducted in Benin and Ghana concluded that most lesions resolve after 8 weeks of treatment.[46,47] In 2010, Nienhuis and colleagues[48] reported the first randomized trial of rifampin plus streptomycin for early limited BU, defined as lesions of less than 6 months' duration comprising nodules or ulcers less than 10 cm in diameter. Rifampin plus streptomycin given daily for 8 weeks, or for 4 weeks, followed by rifampin plus clarithromycin (both oral) daily for 4 weeks, all without surgery, healed BU in more than 90% of patients by 1 year. These results, coupled with experimental data in mice and a case report describing resolution of advanced BU after 8 weeks of rifampin plus clarithromycin,[49] support studies of fully oral, less-toxic regimens, such as rifampin plus clarithromycin or rifapentine plus moxifloxacin.[50]

For advanced BU, rifampin plus streptomycin therapy is under investigation. In a study in the Democratic Republic of Congo, 61 patients with

PCR-positive ulcers (longest diameter>10 cm) were treated with daily rifampin plus streptomycin, treatment was extended to 12 weeks, and surgery was performed 4 weeks after antibiotics treatment was begun; 98% were classified as cured after 2 years.[51] Further studies in patients with large BU lesions, coordinated by the WHO, will aim to determine the best time for surgery within the course of antibiotics.

In some BU lesions, treatment with antibiotics may cause temporary immune-mediated inflammation with clinical worsening, proposed as a paradoxic sign of treatment success.[52] Awareness may prevent unnecessary treatment changes, reduce surgeries, and improve the accuracy of treatment trials.

ACKNOWLEDGMENTS

The authors thank Siripan Phatisawad for making the map.

REFERENCES

1. Silva MT, Portaels F, Pedrosa J. Pathogenetic mechanisms of the intracellular parasite *Mycobacterium ulcerans* leading to Buruli ulcer. Lancet Infect Dis 2009;9:699–710.
2. World Health Organization. Buruli ulcer progress report, 2004–2008. Wkly Epidemiol Rec 2008;83: 145–54.
3. Walsh DS, Eyase F, Onyango D, et al. Short report: clinical and molecular evidence for a case of Buruli ulcer (*Mycobacterium ulcerans* infection) in Kenya. Am J Trop Med Hyg 2009;81:1110–3.
4. Barogui Y, Johnson RC, van der Werf TS, et al. Functional limitations after surgical or antibiotic treatment for Buruli ulcer in Benin. Am J Trop Med Hyg 2009; 81:82–7.
5. McGann H, Stragier P, Portaels F, et al. Buruli ulcer in United Kingdom tourist returning from Latin America. Emerg Infect Dis 2009;15:1827–9.
6. Portaels F, Silva MT, Meyers WM. Buruli ulcer. Clin Dermatol 2009;27:291–305.
7. Marion E, Eyangoh S, Yeramian E, et al. Seasonal and regional dynamics of *M. ulcerans* transmission in environmental context: deciphering the role of water bugs as hosts and vectors. PLoS Negl Trop Dis 2010;4:e731.
8. Johnson PD, Lavender CJ. Correlation between Buruli ulcer and vector-borne notifiable diseases, Victoria, Australia. Emerg Infect Dis 2009;15: 614–5.
9. Durnez L, Suykerbuyk P, Nicolas V, et al. The role of terrestrial small mammals as reservoir of *Mycobacterium ulcerans* in Benin. Appl Environ Microbiol 2010;76:4574–7.
10. Jacobsen KH, Padgett JJ. Risk factors for *Mycobacterium ulcerans* infection. Int J Infect Dis 2010;14: e677–81.
11. Sopoh GE, Barogui YT, Johnson RC, et al. Family relationship, water contact and occurrence of Buruli ulcer in Benin. PLoS Negl Trop Dis 2010; 4:e746.
12. Johnson RC, Nackers F, Glynn JR, et al. Association of HIV infection and *Mycobacterium ulcerans* disease in Benin. AIDS 2008;22:901–3.
13. Portaels F, Aguiar J, Debacker M, et al. *Mycobacterium bovis* BCG vaccination as prophylaxis against *Mycobacterium ulcerans* osteomyelitis in Buruli ulcer disease. Infect Immun 2004;72:62–5.
14. Smith PG, Revill WD, Lukwago E, et al. The protective effect of BCG against *Mycobacterium ulcerans* disease: a controlled trial in an endemic area of Uganda. Trans R Soc Trop Med Hyg 1977;70:449–57.
15. Portaels F, Aguiar J, Debacker M, et al. Prophylactic effect of *Mycobacterium bovis* BCG vaccination against osteomyelitis in children with *Mycobacterium ulcerans* disease (Buruli ulcer). Clin Diagn Lab Immunol 2002;9:1389–91.
16. Nackers F, Dramaix M, Johnson RC, et al. BCG vaccine effectiveness against Buruli ulcer: a case-control study in Benin. Am J Trop Med Hyg 2006; 75:768–74.
17. Huygen K, Adjei O, Affolabi D, et al. Buruli ulcer disease: prospects for a vaccine. Med Microbiol Immunol 2009;198:69–77.
18. Vandelannoote K, Durnez L, Amissah D, et al. Application of real-time PCR in Ghana, a Buruli ulcer-endemic country, confirms the presence of *Mycobacterium ulcerans* in the environment. FEMS Microbiol Lett 2010;304:191–4.
19. Durnez L, Stragier P, Roebben K, et al. A comparison of DNA extraction procedures for the detection of *Mycobacterium ulcerans*, the causative agent of Buruli ulcer, in clinical and environmental specimens. J Microbiol Methods 2008;76:152–8.
20. Portaels F, Meyers WM, Ablordey A, et al. First cultivation and characterization of *Mycobacterium ulcerans* from the environment. PLoS Negl Trop Dis 2008;2: e178.
21. Tobias NJ, Seemann T, Pidot SJ, et al. Mycolactone gene expression is controlled by strong SigA-like promoters with utility in studies of *Mycobacterium ulcerans* and Buruli ulcer. PLoS Negl Trop Dis 2009;3: e553.
22. Demangel C, Stinear TP, Cole ST. Buruli ulcer: reductive evolution enhances pathogenicity of *Mycobacterium ulcerans*. Nat Rev Microbiol 2009;7:50–60.
23. Stragier P, Ablordey A, Bayonne LM, et al. Heterogeneity among *Mycobacterium ulcerans* isolates from Africa. Emerg Infect Dis 2006;12:844–7.
24. Ortiz RH, Leon DA, Estevez HO, et al. Differences in virulence and immune response induced in a murine

model by isolates of *Mycobacterium ulcerans* from different geographic areas. Clin Exp Immunol 2009;157:271–81.

25. Kaser M, Gutmann O, Hauser J, et al. Lack of insertional-deletional polymorphism in a collection of *Mycobacterium ulcerans* isolates from Ghanaian Buruli ulcer patients. J Clin Microbiol 2009;47: 3640–6.

26. Kaser M, Hauser J, Pluschke G. Single nucleotide polymorphisms on the road to strain differentiation in *Mycobacterium ulcerans*. J Clin Microbiol 2009; 47:3647–52.

27. Qi W, Kaser M, Roltgen K, et al. Genomic diversity and evolution of *Mycobacterium ulcerans* revealed by next-generation sequencing. PLoS Pathog 2009;5:e1000580.

28. Roltgen K, Qi W, Ruf MT, et al. Single nucleotide polymorphism typing of *Mycobacterium ulcerans* reveals focal transmission of Buruli ulcer in a highly endemic region of Ghana. PLoS Negl Trop Dis 2010;4:e751.

29. Boulkroun S, Guenin-Mace L, Thoulouze MI, et al. Mycolactone suppresses T cell responsiveness by altering both early signaling and posttranslational events. J Immunol 2010;184:1436–44.

30. Torrado E, Fraga AG, Logarinho E, et al. IFN-gamma-dependent activation of macrophages during experimental infections by *Mycobacterium ulcerans* is impaired by the toxin mycolactone. J Immunol 2010;184:947–55.

31. Hong H, Coutanceau E, Leclerc M, et al. Mycolactone diffuses from *Mycobacterium ulcerans*-infected tissues and targets mononuclear cells in peripheral blood and lymphoid organs. PLoS Negl Trop Dis 2008;2:e325.

32. Phillips R, Sarfo FS, Guenin-Mace L, et al. Immunosuppressive signature of cutaneous *Mycobacterium ulcerans* infection in the peripheral blood of patients with Buruli ulcer disease. J Infect Dis 2009;200: 1675–84.

33. Kiszewski AE, Becerril E, Aguilar LD, et al. The local immune response in ulcerative lesions of Buruli disease. Clin Exp Immunol 2006;143:445–51.

34. Schutte D, Pluschke G. Immunosuppression and treatment-associated inflammatory response in patients with *Mycobacterium ulcerans* infection (Buruli ulcer). Expert Opin Biol Ther 2009;9: 187–200.

35. Stanford JL, Revill WD, Gunthorpe WJ, et al. The production and preliminary investigation of Burulin, a new skin test reagent for *Mycobacterium ulcerans* infection. J Hyg (Lond) 1975;74:7–16.

36. Phanzu MD, Bafende AE, Imposo BB, et al. Undertreated necrotizing fasciitis masquerading as ulcerated edematous *Mycobacterium ulcerans* infection (Buruli ulcer). Am J Trop Med Hyg 2010;82: 478–81.

37. Beissner M, Herbinger KH, Bretzel G. Laboratory diagnosis of Buruli ulcer disease. Future Microbiol 2010;5:363–70.

38. Herbinger KH, Adjei O, Awua-Boateng NY, et al. Comparative study of the sensitivity of different diagnostic methods for the laboratory diagnosis of Buruli ulcer disease. Clin Infect Dis 2009;48:1055–64.

39. Stragier P, Ablordey A, Durnez L, et al. VNTR analysis differentiates *Mycobacterium ulcerans* and IS2404 positive mycobacteria. Syst Appl Microbiol 2007;30:525–30.

40. Sarfo FS, Phillips RO, Rangers B, et al. Detection of mycolactone A/B in *Mycobacterium ulcerans*-infected human tissue. PLoS Negl Trop Dis 2010;4: e577.

41. O'Brien DP, Hughes AJ, Cheng AC, et al. Outcomes for *Mycobacterium ulcerans* infection with combined surgery and antibiotic therapy: findings from a south-eastern Australian case series. Med J Aust 2007;186:58–61.

42. Schunk M, Thompson W, Klutse E, et al. Outcome of patients with Buruli ulcer after surgical treatment with or without antimycobacterial treatment in Ghana. Am J Trop Med Hyg 2009;81:75–81.

43. Junghanss T, Um Boock A, Vogel M, et al. Phase change material for thermotherapy of Buruli ulcer: a prospective observational single centre proof-of-principle trial. PLoS Negl Trop Dis 2009;3:e380.

44. Etuaful S, Carbonnelle B, Grosset J, et al. Efficacy of the combination rifampin-streptomycin in preventing growth of *Mycobacterium ulcerans* in early lesions of Buruli ulcer in humans. Antimicrob Agents Chemother 2005;49:3182–6.

45. World Health Organization. Provisional guidance on the role of specific antibiotics in the management of *Mycobacterium ulcerans* disease (Buruli ulcer). (WHO/CDS/CPE/GBUI/2004). Geneva (Switzerland): World Health Organization; 2004.

46. Chauty A, Ardant MF, Adeye A, et al. Promising clinical efficacy of streptomycin-rifampin combination for treatment of Buruli ulcer (*Mycobacterium ulcerans* disease). Antimicrob Agents Chemother 2007; 51:4029–35.

47. Sarfo FS, Phillips R, Asiedu K, et al. The clinical efficacy of combination of rifampin and streptomycin for treatment of *Mycobacterium ulcerans* disease. Antimicrob Agents Chemother 2010;54: 3678–85.

48. Nienhuis WA, Stienstra Y, Thompson WA, et al. Antimicrobial treatment for early, limited *Mycobacterium ulcerans* infection: a randomised controlled trial. Lancet 2010;375:664–72.

49. Dossou AD, Sopoh GE, Johnson CR, et al. Management of *Mycobacterium ulcerans* infection in a pregnant woman in Benin using rifampicin and clarithromycin. Med J Aust 2008;189:532–3.

50. Ji B, Chauffour A, Robert J, et al. Bactericidal and sterilizing activities of several orally administered combined regimens against *Mycobacterium ulcerans* in mice. Antimicrob Agents Chemother 2008;52:1912–6.

51. Kibadi K, Boelaert M, Fraga AG, et al. Response to treatment in a prospective cohort of patients with large ulcerated lesions suspected to be Buruli ulcer (*Mycobacterium ulcerans* disease). PLoS Negl Trop Dis 2010;4:e736.

52. O'Brien DP, Robson ME, Callan PP, et al. "Paradoxical" immune-mediated reactions to *Mycobacterium ulcerans* during antibiotic treatment: a result of treatment success, not failure. Med J Aust 2009;191: 564–6.

Outbreak of Nontuberculous Mycobacterial Disease in the Central Pacific

Joseph V. Lillis, MD[a],*, David Ansdell, BA[b]

KEYWORDS

- Mycobacterium marinum • Nontuberculous mycobacteria
- Pacific islanders

Approximately 10% of the island population of Satowan (population, 650 persons), a small, remote coral island in the central Pacific, suffers from an acquired, chronic, disfiguring skin condition known locally as "spam." This skin disease has affected the island population since shortly after World War II. An investigation in 2007 revealed that this skin disease is caused by a nontuberculous mycobacterial infection (NTM) closely related to *Mycobacterium marinum*.[1] This article reviews the fascinating history of this skin disease on Satowan, its distinctive clinical presentation, and recommendations for diagnosis and treatment of clinically similar skin lesions in Pacific Islanders.

GEOGRAPHY AND HISTORY OF THE ISLAND

Satowan is one of the 607 islands in the Federated States of Micronesia (FSM), an independent, sovereign nation that extends 1800 miles (2900 km) across the Caroline Islands in the central Pacific, east of the Philippines and south of Guam. FSM comprises the four states of Kosrae, Pohnpei, Chuuk and Yap. Our story takes place in a sparsely populated, outer island cluster of atolls in the southeastern part of Chuuk, known as the Mortlock Islands. Satowan is the main islet of Satowan Atoll, one of four atolls in the Mortlocks. Two hundred miles from Chuuk's

population center in Weno, the indigenous Micronesians of the 1.1-km^2 island of Satowan have survived for centuries, living mostly a subsistence lifestyle with a diet composed of local marine life and the bounty of crops brought by their voyaging ancestors. These introduced plants provide the staple foods of breadfruit, coconut, and taro.

The Caroline Islands were likely settled by people originating from Southeast Asia around 3000 BC. In the sixteenth century, Magellan and subsequent Spanish explorers claimed this part of the Pacific Ocean for Spain, but most of these remote islands were largely ignored by the outside world until the nineteeenth century when they were visited by whalers, traders, and missionaries from Europe, the United States, and Japan. In 1898, the Spanish empire collapsed and Germany purchased many of Spain's holdings in Micronesia. Germany had economic goals and developed local resources of copra (dried coconut meat) and guano (accumulated droppings of seabirds, from which commercial phosphates were extracted).[2] Although claimed by European nations for more than 300 years, the central Pacific islands remained, for all practical purposes, uncolonized. That changed in October of 1914, when Japan seized Palau, Saipan, Pohnpei, Kosrae, Chuuk, and Yap from Germany at the beginning of World War I.[2] Unlike Spain and Germany, whose interests in the islands were largely economic, Japan looked at them as an

[a] Division of Dermatology, Department of Medicine, University of California, San Diego Medical Center, Suite 2A, 3rd floor, 4168 Front Street, #8675, San Diego, CA 92103, USA
[b] John A. Burns School of Medicine, University of Hawai, 651 Ilalo Street, Medical Education Building Honolulu, HI 96813, USA
* Corresponding author.
E-mail address: jlillis01@gmail.com

Dermatol Clin 29 (2011) 9–13
doi:10.1016/j.det.2010.09.008
0733-8635/11/$ – see front matter © 2011 Elsevier Inc. All rights reserved.

derm.theclinics.com

integral part of a growing empire. In addition to investing resources into roads, harbors, communications systems, and transportation facilities, Japan encouraged its citizens to colonize the islands. From 1920 to 1942, the population of Japanese living on the islands of the central Pacific grew from approximately 3000 to over 93,000.[3] Although half of these colonial Japanese were on Saipan, by 1942 there were nearly 5000 living in Chuuk as well.[3]

Along with the influx of Japanese families came an influx of Japanese culture. Japanese-style homes and markets were built and traditional island agriculture was replaced by Japanese crops and domesticated animals. One of the hindrances to living on these tropical islands was the abundance of mosquitoes, which bred in pools of fresh and brackish water. To counter the mosquitoes, the Japanese introduced small fresh water fish called medaka (*Oryzias latipes*) to many islands, including Satowan. Surviving in small collections of standing water, medaka ate mosquito larvae and helped control local mosquito populations (Kino S. Ruben, Medical Officer, Chuuk Department of Health, personal communication, June 2007).

In the years leading up to World War II, Japan's intentions in the region shifted from economic development and colonization to military transformation as they established military bases throughout the central Pacific. Chuuk's main population center in Chuuk Lagoon (then known as Truk Lagoon) comprises a tight cluster of high volcanic islands surrounded by a 50-km wide lagoon that, in turn, is surrounded by a circumferential, halo-like protective coral reef. This unique geography made Truk Lagoon an ideal maritime stronghold for the Japanese fleet. Known as the Fourth Base Force (*konkyochitai*), Truk soon became the forward anchorage for all Japanese naval garrisons in the Eastern Caroline Islands.[2] Smaller, outer islands were also used by the Japanese military. As the widest strip of land in the Mortlock Islands, Satowan was an ideal location for a small, remote airbase. Construction began in 1943 after residents of Satowan were forced to move to Kutu and Moch, two smaller islets on Satowan Atoll.[4] A concrete runway and other military installations were built, transforming Satowan into Japan's largest military base in the Mortlock Islands.

On February 17, 1944, a United States carrier fleet began a now historic 2-day bombing of Truk Lagoon in a mission known as Operation Hailstone. Forty-five Japanese ships and 275 Japanese aircraft were destroyed and another 27 vessels were damaged, essentially removing Truk lagoon as a major threat to Allied island-hopping operations

in the central Pacific.[2] Allied forces then disabled Japanese installations elsewhere in the Carolines and reclaimed control of the central Pacific. Nevertheless on April 30, 1944, eight US destroyers and nine cruisers bombarded Satowan with 1400 rounds of 5-inch shells and 800 rounds of 8-inch shells, destroying the runway and surrounding military installations.[5,6] Although the bombardment met with no opposition and is described by some historians as a "training exercise"[5] or "target practice"[6] before Allied invasions of islands closer to Japan, the bombing was so extensive that it created large bomb craters in the center of the island.

After the bombing, Satowan residents returned from Kutu and Moch to find their island transformed by Japanese military occupation and the subsequent American bombardment. In 1947, the Caroline Islands, now free from Japan's occupation, became part of the US-governed Trust Territory of the Pacific. American foods, such as Spam, soon became a regular part of the Micronesian's diet.

In the decades that followed, as they replanted taro fields, breadfruit trees, and coconut palms, the Satowanese began to observe an odd skin disease; they could neither attribute a cause to it nor find an effective treatment (**Fig. 1**). Local health officials began to refer to it as "island psoriasis," and residents began to refer to it as "spam," after the processed

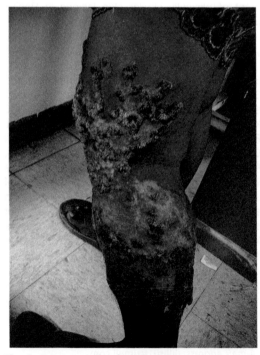

Fig. 1. Representative lesions. Large, verrucous plaques on leg of patient from Satowan (Chuuk, FSM).

food product that the skin lesions were said to resemble. Treatments included bleach, battery acid, cigarette burns, hot ashes, electrocautery, and surgical excision and were usually ineffective, resulting only in disease recurrence and disfigurement (Kino S. Ruben, Medical Officer, Chuuk Department of Health, personal communication, June 2007).

INVESTIGATION

In the summer of 2004, health officials from the FSM reported this epidemic on Satowan to the Tripler Army Medical Center on O'ahu hoping to find a definitive cause, an effective treatment, and a successful prevention strategy. Histopathologic specimens were obtained and reviewed, but no definitive diagnosis established. Two years later, the Polynesian Voyaging Society announced plans to sail traditional voyaging canoes from Hawai'i to Japan via Micronesia. In a partnership with Aloha Medical Mission (AMM), a series of medical clinics were organized in Micronesia to coincide with the arrival of the sailing canoes. Prior to departure, members of the AMM were contacted by the Hawai'i Department of Health and asked to further investigate this mysterious illness that had afflicted inhabitants of Satowan since World War II. While in Weno, Chuuk's capital city, six affected Satowanese islanders were evaluated by members of the AMM, but tissue cultures were negative and histopathologic analysis was again inconclusive.

Around the same time, in the fall of 2006, a 29-year-old man from Satowan presented to an indigent care clinic in Portland, Oregon, with an 18-year history of enlarging verrucous plaques on his left lower extremity that started when he lived on Satowan (**Fig. 2**). A tissue culture demonstrated *M marinum*.[7] Consistent with previous reports from Chuuk health officials in 2004, he estimated that 10% of the people on his home island had similar lesions. In the summer of 2007, an outbreak investigation was initiated with local health aides on Satowan to determine the causative organism and potential risk factors for developing the condition. Thirty-nine cases of verrucous plaques greater than 3 cm in size and present for more than three months were identified, with the majority (74%) in males. The median age was 26.0 years, the mean duration of involvement was 12.5 years, and the longest period of involvement was 53 years. All but one case involved the upper or lower extremities, and the most frequently affected area was the knee (44%).[1]

On histopathologic analysis, all biopsies contained findings typical of NTM or deep fungal infections (**Fig. 3**), but stains for mycobacterial and fungal organism were negative as were

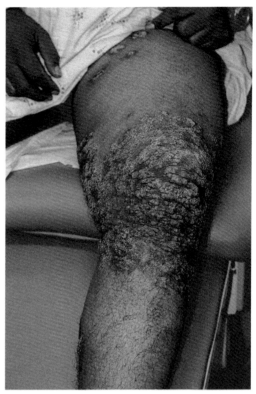

Fig. 2. Index case from Satowanese patient who was evaluated while he was living in Portland, OR.

all tissue cultures. Polymerase chain reaction (PCR) evaluation was positive for NTM and the PCR product sequences had close identity with *M marinum*. One important risk factor was taro farming, which involves many hours of kneeling or squatting in standing water. Another significant

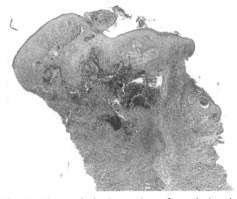

Fig. 3. Histopathologic sections from lesional skin demonstrating irregular epidermal and follicular hyperplasia with a dense, nodular, mixed infiltrate consisting of epithelioid histiocytes, neutrophils, eosinophils, lymphocytes, and plasma cells with a thickened and fibrotic papillary dermis.

risk factor was contact with large water-filled depressions in the center of the island (**Fig. 4**). These water-filled depressions, created by the extensive bombing in World War II, contained large numbers of small fish, identified as the medaka (*Oryzias latipes*), that the Japanese introduced a half-century earlier.

Due to the limited resources available, most Satowanese patients were treated with 3 months of monotherapy with doxycycline. Treatment results were mixed. Those with limited involvement responded well, but those with more extensive involvement had incomplete treatment or disease recurrence.

DISCUSSION

Satowan residents have believed for many years that the skin condition is related in some way to the Japanese occupation before World War II (Kino S. Ruben, Medical Officer, Chuuk Department of Health, personal communication, June 2007). The investigation in 2007 may support this long-held belief. PCR analysis and culture from the index case demonstrate the presence of a NTM closely related to *M marinum*. *M marinum* is known to cause disease in humans through aquatic exposure of traumatized skin, and the investigation points to the water-filled bomb craters as a likely source of infection. Within these water-filled bomb craters, medaka, a fish native to Japan, not the Pacific Islands,[8] survives in abundance without any visible sign of infection. This species of fish, when compared with other species used in laboratory study of mycobacterial diseases, can tolerate chronic infection with *M marinum* without outward signs of infection.[9] Thus, the introduction of healthy-appearing medaka to Satowan to control the mosquito populations may have also introduced an organism

closely related to *M marinum*. After the island environment was altered by bombing and the bomb craters filled with water, an ideal environment was created for the proliferation of the organism. Then, as island residents began to swim or bathe in these pools of water, the organism had direct contact with traumatized skin, thus explaining the large numbers of cases seen after World War II.

Since the 2007 investigation, 24 additional cases have been identified on Satowan (review of photographs of skin lesions on Satowanese patients who were not examined during the initial investigation, August 2009), bringing the total to 63, which is approximately the 10% figure estimated in the original health report. In addition, similar cases with no connection to Satowan, have been described. In 1998, two cases were reported in patients from Nauru and one from Western Samoa, both islands in the south Pacific.[10] All three cases had cultures positive for *M marinum* and were successfully treated with a 3-month course of rifampin and trimethoprim-sulfamethoxazole. Additionally, in 2008 there was an unpublished, culture-negative, case in Hawai'i with similar clinical and histologic findings to the patients from Satowan that completely resolved when treated with doxycycline (**Fig. 5**). This patient developed her lesions while living on Houk, a small outer island in western Chuuk, which contains a central freshwater lake. She reported other people on her island that were similarly affected. Due to the difficulty in growing the organism in culture and its unusual clinical presentation, other cases of this condition may exist as well, possibly misdiagnosed as culture-negative chromoblastomycosis or tuberculosis cutis verrucosa.

Although this distinct disease presentation does not seem to be limited to residents of Satowan, it does seem to be limited to Pacific Islanders. The

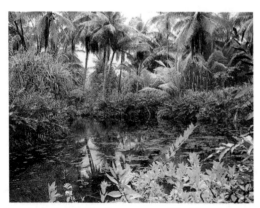

Fig. 4. One of two large water-filled bomb crater lakes in the center of Satowan (Chuuk, FSM) where people swim and bathe.

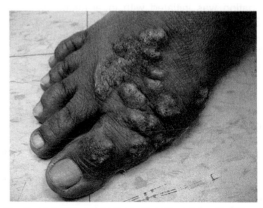

Fig. 5. Lesion on right foot of patient from the island of Houk (Chuuk, FSM).

reason for this is uncertain. It may be due to a chronic environmental exposure, a genetic susceptibility, coinfection with another unidentified organism, and/or a particularly virulent strain of NTM seen only in the Pacific. It may also simply be due to long-standing, untreated disease; something for which medically underserved Pacific Islanders are at particular risk.

In a Pacific Islander who presents with chronic, large, verrucous plaques, in which the differential diagnosis includes such conditions as chromoblastomycosis and tuberculosis cutis verrucosa, it is important to consider the diagnosis of a chronic NTM infection. A proper work-up should include biopsies for histopathology and tissue culture, with specific instructions to culture for slow growing NTM, such as *M marinum*. PCR can determine the presence of NTM, but is unable, at this time, to differentiate specific species. Although there is no consensus for treatment, it seems that these patients require empiric, multi-drug antibiotic therapy, especially when presenting with large lesions. Rifampin, in combination with ethambutol, trimethprim-sulfamethoxazole, clarithromycin or minocycline should be started and continued for at least 3 months.[11] If lesions are small and resources are limited, a 3-month treatment course with doxycycline could be considered as well. If lesions recur, however, additional culture and sensitivity testing should govern further multidrug antibiotic therapy.

Unfortunately, the remoteness of Satowan makes additional study and follow-up difficult. Further microbiologic assessment is needed to specifically identify the causative NTM organism and environmental samples are needed from Satowan to further establish the infectious sources on the island. In addition, an investigation on Houk is warranted as well. It seems that this condition is easier to treat when skin lesions are small, so early identification and treatment may be the most cost-effective way of preventing the large disfiguring plaques associated with longstanding infection. Over time, it will be important to determine if limiting exposure of open skin to the water-filled bomb craters and taro fields will prevent new cases.

The introduction of medaka by the Japanese and the extensive bombing by the United States military caused significant environmental changes on Satowan both before and during World War II. These changes may offer an explanation for the sudden appearance of this skin condition after the war. And, although the story of its origin may be unique to Satowan, this distinct presentation of NTM infection affects other Pacific Islanders as well. In any Pacific Islander with large, chronic, progressive verrucous plaques, a proper diagnostic work-up and early, appropriate antibiotic therapy provide the key to preventing large disfiguring plaques like those that have affected the Satowanese for many years.

REFERENCES

1. Lillis JV, Ansdell VE, Ruben K, et al. Sequelae of World War II: an outbreak of chronic cutaneous nontuberculous mycobacterial infection among Satowanese islanders. Clin Infect Dis. 2009;48(11):1541–6.
2. Bailey DE. World War II wrecks of the truk lagoon. Redding (CA): North Valley Diver Publications; 2000. p. 8–17, 165, 188.
3. Peattie MR. Nan'Yo: the rise and fall of the Japanese in Micronesia, 1885–1945. Honolulu (HI): University of Hawai'I Press; 1988. p. 160–1.
4. Poyer L, Falgout S, Carucci LM. The typhoon of war: micronesian experiences of the Pacific war. Honolulu (HI): University of Hawai'i Press; 2001. p. 88–9.
5. Morison SE. New Guinea and the Marianas, March 1944-August 1944. History of United States naval operations in World War II, vol. 8. Champaign (IL): University of Illinois Press; 2001. p. 40–1.
6. Karig W. Battle report—the end of an empire. Council on Books in Wartime. New York: Farrar & Rinehart; 1944. p. 197–8.
7. Lillis JV, Winthrop KL, White CR, et al. Mycobacterium marinum presenting as large verrucous plaques on the lower extremity of a South Pacific Islander. Am J Trop Med Hyg 2008;79(2):166–7.
8. Parenti LR. A phylogenetic analysis and taxonomic revision of ricefishes, *Oryzias* and relatives (Beloniformes, Adrianichthyidae). Zool J Linn Soc 2008; 154:494–610.
9. Broussard GW, Ennis DG. Mycobacterium marinum produces long-term chronic infections in medaka: a new animal model for studying human tuberculosis. Comp Biochem Physiol C Toxicol Pharmacol 2007;145(1):45–54.
10. Lee MW, Brenan J. Mycobacterium marinum: chronic and extensive infections of the lower limbs in South Pacific Islanders. Australas J Dermatol 1998;39:173–6.
11. Rallis E, Koumantaki-Mathioudaki E. Treatment of Mycobacterium marinum cutaneous infections. Expert Opin Pharmacother 2007;8(17):2965–78.

Dermatology Aboard the USNS *COMFORT*: Disaster Relief Operations in Haiti After the 2010 Earthquake

Kenneth Galeckas, MD[a,b],*

KEYWORDS

- Haiti • Dermatology • Disaster relief
- Planned humanitarian assistance mission

On the 12th of January 2010, Haiti was struck by a 7.0 Richter magnitude earthquake that devastated its already fragile capital region. Approximately 230,000[1] people died either immediately or during ensuing weeks, mostly due to acute trauma. Countless others suffered significant life- or limb-threatening injuries. As a part of the United States' response to this tragedy, eventually named Operation Unified Response (OUR), the United States Navy deployed hundreds of physicians and other medical response individuals on the USNS *Comfort*, a US Navy hospital ship based in Baltimore, Maryland. OUR was a military joint task force operation that was augmented by both governmental and nongovernmental organizations (eg, US Agency for International Development, Project HOPE, and Operation Smile). Our mission was to bring urgently needed medical and logistical support to the region. I had the distinct privilege to serve as the dermatologist for this mission.

The *Comfort* (**Fig. 1**) is one of two *Mercy* class hospital ships operated by the US Navy. The *Comfort* and its West Coast counterpart, USNS *Mercy*, participate in biennial humanitarian missions that bring health care to many developing nations in Central and South America and along the Pacific Rim. In addition, these ships are on perpetual standby as part of the national response to natural disasters, both in the United States and abroad. Recent disaster-related missions have included deployments to New Orleans after Hurricane Katrina and to Indonesia after the 2004 tsunami. Although most missions render humanitarian assistance or disaster relief, the *Comfort* also provided combat medical support for Operation Desert Shield and Operation Desert Storm. In this instance, most of the reporting personnel received less than 24 hours notice to prepare for deployment, get to Baltimore, and report aboard. The *Comfort* set sail on January 16, 2010, with more than 1000 medical and support staff. It arrived in Port-au-Prince and was receiving her first patients within 7 days of the earthquake.

Commissioned in 1987, the *Comfort*'s capabilities are impressive. It was originally built and launched as an oil tanker, the SS *Rose City*, in 1976. At 892 feet, almost as long as an aircraft carrier, it boasts a 50-bed trauma emergency room, 12 operating rooms, a 20-bed recovery room, a 30-bed intensive care unit, 400

The views expressed in this article are those of the author and do not necessarily reflect the official policy or position of the Department of the Navy, Department of Defense, or the US Government.

[a] Department of Dermatology, National Naval Medical Center, 8901 Wisconsin Avenue, Bethesda, MD 20889, USA
[b] Uniformed Services University of the Health Sciences, 4301 Jones Bridge Road, Bethesda, MD 20814, USA
* Department of Dermatology, National Naval Medical Center, 8901 Wisconsin Avenue, Bethesda, MD 20889.
E-mail address: kenneth.galeckas@med.navy.mil

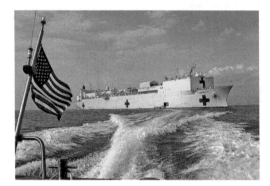

Fig. 1. The USNS *Comfort*, at anchor off Port-au-Prince, Haiti, February 2010.

intermediate-care beds, 500 minimal-care beds, and full radiologic and laboratory support. For this mission, the ship was staffed with many medical and surgical subspecialty physicians (**Table 1**).[2]

OUR was designed as a disaster relief operation. This mission's purpose was distinctly different from a carefully planned humanitarian assistance mission (HAM). HAMs are preceded by site visits in an effort to efficiently coordinate care once the *Comfort* arrives on schedule at a particular location. On typical ship-based HAMs, the dermatologist goes ashore to set up clinics that have been announced to the local population. Usually, these announcements encourage hundreds of people to seek care. In this way, there is a virtually endless stream of patients and the care that is provided is limited only by time and supplies. The Haitian earthquake destroyed nearly all of Port-au-Prince's piers; thus, the *Comfort* anchored farther out in the harbor, which in turn made helicopters and small boats necessary to transfer patients. Because of the orthopedic nature of many injuries, transportation of patients required stretchers and many stretcher-bearers. As such, helicopters and small boats filled quickly with seriously injured patients, thereby limiting my ability to obtain transportation to land.

When traveling to local hospitals, our teams of physicians and support staff were assigned security escorts, thereby adding another layer of

Table 1
Breakdown of physician/staff specialties aboard *USNS Comfort* for Operation Unified Response Haiti

USNS *Comfort* for OUR Haiti—2010[a]

Physician Staff			
Anesthesiology	11	Neurology (pediatrics)	1
Cardiology	1	Neurosurgery	2
Critical care	3	Obstetrics/gynecology	2
Dermatology	1	Opthalmology	3
Develomental pediatrics	1	Oral/maxillofacial surgery	1
Emergency medicine	5	Orthopedic surgery	12
Emergency medicine (pediatrics)	1	Orthopedic surgery (pediatrics)	1
Endocrinology (pediatrics)	1	Otolaryngology	1
Family practice	4	Pediatrics	4
Gastroenterology	1	Plastic surgery	1
General surgery	2	Psychiatry	1
Infectious disease	2	Radiology	4
Internal medicine	2	Urology	2
Nephrology	2	Vascular surgery	1
Neurology	1	Wound care	1
Nonphysician Clinical Staff			
Dentist	3	Optometry	2
Nurse anesthetist	13	Clinical psychology	2
Family nurse practitioner	3	Social worker	2
Medical/surgical nursing	165	Wound care nurse practitioner	2

[a] Includes volunteer nonmilitary staff augmentees.

Data from Amundson D, Dadekian G, Etienne M, et al. Practicing internal medicine onboard the USNS COMFORT in the aftermath of the Haitian earthquake. Ann Intern Med 2010;152(11):733–7.

logistical complexity. In the 2 months after the earthquake, the crowds were peaceful and were welcoming, likely the result of the general goodwill cultivated from the *Comfort*'s previous missions to Haiti, most recently as part of Operation Continuing Promise in the spring of 2009. The *Comfort* and other US Navy ships delivering humanitarian assistance have been frequent visitors to Haiti for many years. As a testament to the US Navy's previous efforts, Haiti's Ministry of Health specifically requested the *Comfort* to be dispatched to Haiti after the earthquake.

As the initial surge of trauma waned over several weeks, I was able to go ashore and make several trips to local hospitals, orphanages, and schools that had been converted into makeshift clinics. My first trip ashore was to a local children's hospital as part of a team that had a mission to establish a relationship with the staff and see how we could be of service. Knowing I was a dermatologist, the hospital's doctors showed me several patients with scabies, head lice, and tinea capitis. Those conditions were commonplace and likely exacerbated by overcrowding and chronic sanitation issues. Because of my limited opportunity to go ashore, I quickly developed and disseminated a protocol on how to send teledermatology consults to the *Comfort* to help assist local physicians with difficult dermatologic cases. Every time a medical team went ashore, I sent along copies of my teledermatology protocol to be distributed to the local health workers. Because the e-mail address was disseminated widely, my services as a dermatologist were called on often. For most teledermatology cases, the diagnosis was straightforward. The major hurdle was whether or not the consulting clinician had appropriate medicines to treat the patient.

Dermatologic complaints encompassed approximately 25% of all acute visits to the *Comfort's* sickbay, which is a 6-bed shipboard clinic that provides care for the large crew (more than 1200 people at times). Most patients presented with allergic and/or irritant contact dermatitis or dermatophyte infections. The tinea infections seen among the ship's crew were brought aboard by most patients—flaring as a result of the long hours, heat, and humidity. There were scattered cases of acne, eczema, warts, and psoriasis. There were several cases of phototoxicity from doxycycline, the antimalarial prophylaxis of choice. Doxycycline was preferred over atovaquone/proguanil (Malarone) or chloroquine because the once-a-day dosing made it easy for ship's company to take at daily muster.

For me, the most interesting cases were the incidental diagnoses of several Haitian patients who were admitted with earthquake-related traumatic injuries. Below are the stories of two such individuals:

Patient #1: I was asked to see JD, an approximately 9-year-old boy (aged based on dental examination), for skin lesions (**Fig. 2**A). This young boy was abandoned by his parents and left on the doorstep of an orphanage shortly after the earthquake. An orphanage volunteer brought him to the ship to treat what was thought to be a traumatic eye injury. His right eye appeared quite swollen with overlying erosions and ulcerations. I found that he was malnourished and clearly suffered from a developmental or neurologic disability. Skin examination was significant for abundant

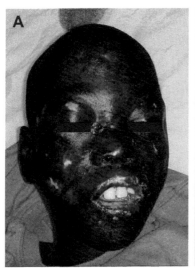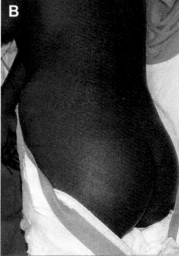

Fig. 2. (*A, B*) Nine-year-old boy with XP phenotype. Note the distinct photogradient (*B*).

widespread hyperkeratotic pigmented papules scattered on all sun-exposed areas with a distinct photogradient. Double-covered areas showed minimal to no damage (see Fig. 2B). Physical examination showed a xeroderma pigmentosum (XP) phenotype. Biopsy of three hyperkeratotic lesions showed pigmented actinic keratoses. On clinical examination, his eye "injury" was noted to be a solid mass. Biopsy confirmed squamous cell carcinoma, prompting enucleation by an oculoplastic surgeon. After 12 days of postoperative convalescence on the *Comfort*, JD was discharged to a local hospital with the ultimate goal of engaging the Xeroderma Pigmentosum Society for assistance with subsequent care (www.xps.org).

Patient #2: DL was a 7-year-old boy admitted for treatment of a femur fracture. I was consulted for evaluation of skin lesions. He was not accompanied by family on board, which was commonly the case with many of our pediatric patients. On examination, DL was suspicious, hesitant, and uncooperative. I deduced, via a Creole translator, that his skin lesions had been present for a "long time," that that they were getting worse, and they seem to spread with scratching. His sister was affected by similar lesions. He also stated that he is often teased at school because of his skin problem. There were many hypopigmented flat-topped papules scatted about his face, arms and trunk, some in linear arrangements (Fig. 3A). My clinical diagnosis was flat warts. Biopsy of a representative lesion on his dorsal hand revealed the classic smoky-blue cytoplasm seen in virally infected keratinocytes, typical of epidermodysplasia verruciformis (EDV) (see Fig. 3B). Having a similarly affected sibling was consistent with the diagnosis of this autosomal recessive disorder. I also suspected untreated or undiagnosed HIV infection, which subsequent ELISA testing confirmed.

Accompanied by a complete package of information, and after stabilization of his femur fracture, he was discharged to a local hospital. The accepting physicians have been made aware of his diagnosis and plan to run HIV testing on his sister. Happily, DL's father, missing since the earthquake, was located and the family has been at least partially reunited.

The memory of these two cases will stick with me for the rest of my career. I had to reconcile the fact that after these children were discharged from the *Comfort,* it is unlikely that they received the care that I am accustomed to providing in the United States. Unfortunately for both of these patients, they are among countless individuals with chronic undiagnosed medical conditions who have been born into a society with, at best, a struggling medical infrastructure. I am hopeful that local medical care and access to subspecialties will improve as the international community continues its effort to rebuild Haiti.

Questions remain. If the diagnosis of XP had been identified earlier, would protective measures have led to a better outcome? Will this boy succumb to his first melanoma? For the boy with EDV, would antiretroviral therapy have averted the development of socially disabling facial lesions? Without our intervention, when would he have eventually learned that he was HIV positive? Now, with a known underlying diagnosis, perhaps he will not receive well-intentioned but inappropriate treatments. For both patients, how in the world will they practice sun safety in Haiti? With XP, as well as the increased cutaneous carcinogenicity associated with EDV, photoprotection is paramount to long-term survival. I was happy to hear that JD has been sent to the United States and is currently living with a family that has another child with XP. Dr Kenneth Kraemer of the National Institutes of Health,

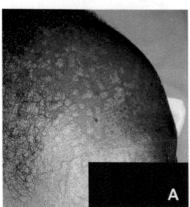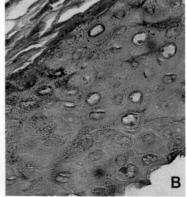

Fig. 3. (*A, B*) Seven-year-old boy with HIV-associated EDV, (*A*) clinical (*B*) histopathology

a pioneer in XP research, was instrumental in coordinating JD's follow-up care.

Although I chronicled only two patients here, 1000 patients were admitted to the *Comfort* in its first 7 weeks in Haiti and each patient has a unique story. Even as the *Comfort*'s mission concludes, the work to rebuild Haiti will continue for years. I encourage all physicians to volunteer their skills to the various volunteer organizations that participate in such humanitarian assistance or disaster relief operations. As echoed by countless clinicians who have been come before me and have been involved in similar endeavors, I have gained as much, if not more, than I gave.

ACKNOWLEDGMENTS

The author would like to sincerely thank Dr Scott Norton for his generous advice, mentorship, and editorial assistance.

REFERENCES

1. USAID Haiti Fact Sheet. July 11, 2010. Available at: www.usaid.giv/helphaiti. Accessed September 17, 2010.
2. Amundson D, Dadekian G, Etienne M, et al. Practicing internal medicine onboard the USNS COMFORT in the aftermath of the Haitian earthquake. Ann Intern Med 2010;152(11):733–7.

Community-associated Methicillin-resistant *Staphylococcus aureus* Skin Infections in the Tropics

Steven Y.C. Tong, MBBS, FRACP, PhD[a,b,]*,
Andrew C. Steer, MBBS, FRACP, PhD[c],
Adam W. Jenney, MBBS, FRACP, PhD[c,d],
Jonathan R. Carapetis, MBBS, FRACP, PhD, MPH[b,e]

KEYWORDS

- Community-associated
- Methicillin-resistant *Staphylococcus aureus* • MRSA
- *Staphylococcus aureus* • Skin and soft tissue infection
- Tropical

Although most of the world's population lives in tropical, developing regions, there has been comparatively little research into the epidemiology of *Staphylococcus aureus* in these areas. The high burden of disease caused by malaria, tuberculosis, and human immunodeficiency virus (HIV) infection, together with a lack of diagnostic microbiology facilities and overall limitations in resource availability, impede understanding of *S aureus* infections. Available data suggest that skin and soft tissue infections (SSTI) caused by *S aureus* are extremely common, particularly in children. In addition, there are high rates of *S aureus* infection in sterile sites (invasive infection) in these same regions, and SSTI are an important source of invasive infection.[1] The understanding that strains of community-associated methicillin-resistant *S aureus* (CA-MRSA) often emerge locally raises the possibility that MRSA is also widespread among populations in the tropics. This review focuses on skin-related manifestations of CA-MRSA in tropical regions and describes what is known about the epidemiology, effects of hygiene and living conditions, diagnosis, and treatment and prevention options at the individual and community levels.

EPIDEMIOLOGY

Most staphylococcal infections involve the skin and soft tissues, and, in tropical regions, such SSTI are abundant. The prevalence of pyoderma, scabies,

ST is supported by an Australian National Health and Medical Research Council Postdoctoral fellowship (436,033). The authors have nothing to disclose.

[a] Tropical and Emerging Infectious Diseases, Menzies School of Health Research, PO Box 41096, Casuarina, Darwin, Northern Territory 0811, Australia
[b] Infectious Diseases Department, Royal Darwin Hospital, 105 Rocklands Drive, Tiwi, Northern Territory 0811, Australia
[c] Centre for International Child Health, Department of Paediatrics, University of Melbourne, Royal Children's Hospital, Flemington Road, Parkville, Melbourne, Victoria 3052, Australia
[d] Infectious Diseases Unit, The Alfred Hospital, 75 Commercial Road, Melbourne, Victoria 3004, Australia
[e] Child Health, Menzies School of Health Research, PO Box 41096, Casuarina, Darwin, Northern Territory 0811, Australia
* Corresponding author. Child Health, Menzies School of Health Research, PO Box 41096, Casuarina, Darwin, Northern Territory 0811, Australia.
E-mail address: Steven.tong@menzies.edu.au

Dermatol Clin 29 (2011) 21–32
doi:10.1016/j.det.2010.09.005

and dermatophyte infections is high,[2] with an estimated 111 million children in developing countries having pyoderma at any one time. Studies from the 1970s found the point prevalence of pyoderma in children to be 7% in Tanzania[3,4] and up to 25% in Panama.[5] The Pacific region has a particularly high prevalence of SSTI. Recent studies in indigenous communities in tropical northern Australia found the point prevalence of pyoderma in children to range from 11% to 20%.[6] In Fiji, the prevalence of pyoderma was 26% in primary school children and 12% in infants.[7] The rates of scabies infection are similarly high, and scabies is a common antecedent for skin infection in these regions.[3,4,6–8] The most common bacterial pathogens of SSTI are Streptococcus pyogenes and S aureus, with recent studies finding recovery rates from swabs of pyoderma lesions of 29% to 80% and 57% to 80% for S pyogenes (group A β-hemolytic streptococci) and S aureus, respectively. Frequently, individual sores are infected with both pathogens.[7,9–11]

These superficial bacterial infections are not always innocuous. Complications include bacteremia[12–14] and other invasive diseases, and, for S pyogenes, the nonsuppurative sequelae of poststreptococcal glomerulonephritis[15] and also possibly acute rheumatic fever.[16] S aureus typically ranks as the third or fourth most commonly isolated bacterial pathogen in surveys of bacteremia in the developing world,[17–21] with skin infections frequently the primary source of the bacteremia.[1,22] Mortality from S aureus bacteremia in low-resource regions is typically high. For example, in a hospital in northeastern Thailand, the case mortality for patients with S aureus sepsis was 52%, causing an estimated 1% of all hospital deaths.[23]

Although S pyogenes remains invariably sensitive to penicillin, antibiotic management for S aureus depends on local rates of antimicrobial resistance. Some experts suggest that if the prevalence of CA-MRSA is greater than 10% in clinical isolates in any given population, then these populations should be considered as high prevalence and β-lactam antibiotics should not be used as empiric therapy for staphylococcal infections.[24] Most studies in tropical regions have been conducted in inpatient hospital settings where rates of methicillin resistance among all S aureus infections range from less than 10% to close to 50%, with most of this attributed to health care–associated (HA) MRSA strains.[25–28] Community-based studies of nasal colonization in India and Brazil found lower rates of MRSA carriage, ranging from 0% to 4%.[29–33]

However, hospital-based studies and colonization data may not reflect the epidemiology of S aureus in community-based SSTI. The few recent studies in tropical and developing country settings that have concentrated on SSTI in outpatients or community-based cohorts showed that CA-MRSA constituted 23% and 11% of S aureus recovered from pyoderma lesions in Australian indigenous[9] and Indian settings[11] respectively, and also 15% of S aureus recovered from SSTI in Hong Kong.[34] Several factors may be contributing to the emergence of CA-MRSA from circulating methicillin-susceptible S aureus (MSSA) strains in less-developed settings; these factors include high rates of secondarily infected scabies, domestic crowding, poor skin hygiene, and the ready availability and use of β-lactam antibiotics.[12,35] In support of this, detailed molecular studies have shown that strains of MSSA acquire the resistance determinant mecA, carried on SCCmec, much more frequently than was previously appreciated.[36]

Nowhere has the problem of CA-MRSA been so striking as in the United States, where CA-MRSA infections have become more common than health care–associated MRSA (HA-MRSA) infections. For example, in San Francisco, the incidence of all types of CA-MRSA infections in 2005 was 316 per 100,000 population, compared with 31 cases of HA-MRSA infections per 100,000.[37] This increase is the direct result of a prevalent strain of CA-MRSA, the USA300 strain.[38–41]

Unlike in the United States, tropical regions have observed a diversity of circulating CA-MRSA clones (**Table 1**).[9,34,42–52] Different clones are typically distinguished by established genotyping techniques such as pulsed-field gel electrophoresis or multilocus sequence typing (MLST). Using MLST, which involves sequencing the internal

Table 1
Dominant clones of CA-MRSA in tropical regions as determined by multilocus sequence typing

Region	Clone	References
East and southeast Asia	ST30, ST59, ST834	34,42–44
Australia (tropical) and Pacific islands	ST93, ST30, CC75, ST8 (USA300) in Hawaii	9,45–47
Subcontinent (India and Pakistan)	ST772	48
Africa	ST88, ST5, ST30, ST80	49–51
Latin America	ST8 (USA300)	52

Abbreviation: ST, sequence type.

fragments of 7 housekeeping genes, S aureus has been shown to be a species with distinct clonal lineages or clonal complexes. Many clones can be found across different continents and include clonal complexes (CC) 30, 8, 45, 15, 5, and 1. However, the proportional representation of these clones varies according to geography. For example, CC30 is common in Singapore and Hong Kong,[44,53] and CC93 is the most prevalent clone of hospital-based isolates in northern Australia.[45]

Perhaps most intriguing is a phylogenetically divergent clone called CC75, which occurs mainly in the tropics.[46] Despite the extensive characterization of S aureus in developed countries, CC75 has to date only been reported in the literature in northern Australia and Cambodia.[9,45,46,54] In addition, analysis of the S aureus multilocus sequence type (MLST) database (http://saureus.mlst.net/) reveals isolates with CC75 alleles from Malaysia, Indonesia, and, somewhat incongruously, Ireland and the Czech Republic. We have also found CC75 in Fiji.[55] CC75 is a phylogenetic outlier whose presence may be related to crowded living conditions, poor skin hygiene, and frequent skin infections.

Several virulence factors have been identified in CA-MRSA isolates,[56] most notably Panton-Valentine leukocidin (PVL). This bicomponent toxin can form pores in the cell membrane of host leukocytes. Early epidemiologic studies linked PVL with cutaneous abscesses, severe SSTI, and necrotizing pneumonia.[57,58] However, controversy exists as to the exact role of PVL. It was not associated with worse outcomes in a multicountry study of complicated SSTI,[59] nor in a Thai study of bacteremic patients.[60] There are also conflicting results regarding the role of PVL from studies using mouse models of SSTI.[61–63] Several recent independent clinical studies in Australia and New Zealand have shown a significant association between PVL and cutaneous furunculosis or skin and soft tissue abscesses.[45,64,65] PVL is also expressed frequently in MSSA isolates; approximately 50% of MSSA isolates from Africa and northern Australia harbor the pvl genes.[45,66] Thus, MSSA is likely to be a significant, but under-recognized, contributor to the burden of PVL disease in these settings.

In summary, evidence suggests that S aureus—related SSTI produces a significant burden of disease in tropical communities. Up to 25% of staphylococcal isolates are CA-MRSA, and ecological conditions favor the emergence and spread of resistance. Of concern, a considerable proportion of both CA-MRSA and MSSA strains causing SSTI harbor the PVL gene, which may cause more severe clinical manifestations.

PREDISPOSING FACTORS

Perhaps the most important predisposing factor for SSTI in tropical zones is the presence of scabies infestation (ie, epidermal infestation by the mite, Sarcoptes scabiei). Scabies lesions that are secondarily infected by S pyogenes or S aureus are very common in many tropical settings. For example, in Fiji, 57% of infants and 30% of children with scabies had evidence of secondary bacterial infection.[7] A reduction in the prevalence of scabies can lead to a reduction in the prevalence of impetigo. This reduction was clearly shown in Panama after mass drug administration program for scabies with permethrin cream, where the prevalence of impetigo was reduced from 32% to 2%. Similarly, in the Solomon Islands after mass drug administration with oral ivermectin, the prevalence of impetigo was reduced from 40% to 21%.[67,68] In addition, community-based treatment of scabies with permethrin in an indigenous Australian community led to a reduction in scabies prevalence from 28.8% to less than 10%. This treatment resulted in a sustained 2-year reduction in impetigo prevalence in children from 69% to less than 35%, with residual impetigo in children being less severe (fewer purulent and crusted lesions).[69]

Overcrowding, poor hygiene, limited water supply, and hot, humid weather have all been linked to SSTI in tropical zones.[4,70] These factors reflect the important role that low socioeconomic status plays; in the main, SSTI in tropical zones is a disease of poverty. Overcrowding is important because of the close personal contact required for transmission of S pyogenes, S aureus, and scabies.[71,72] Washing with water seems to play an important role in the prevention of impetigo. A randomized controlled trial of handwashing promotion and plain soap in Pakistan found a reduction in the incidence of impetigo amongst children of 34% in the intervention group.[73] Antibacterial soap did not provide an advantage compared with plain soap, suggesting that the cleansing process with water is the key factor. This conclusion was supported by a further study in an Australian aboriginal community in which access to a swimming pool was associated with a reduction in the prevalence of impetigo in children, from 62% to 18%.[74]

DIAGNOSIS

Unless there are clinical features that suggest unusual pathogens, most cases of impetigo and furunculosis are caused by S pyogenes or S aureus, or sometimes both. Knowledge of the local antimicrobial resistance pattern of S aureus helps to determine whether culturing such lesions will be clinically useful. In resource-poor regions, there is likely to be limited benefit to routine culture of such lesions if rates of MRSA are low. In regions with higher rates of MRSA, clinicians must consider whether to culture infected lesions, or whether changing the empirical therapy away from β-lactams will be more effective.

Point-of-care rapid diagnostics to determine whether MRSA or PVL-producing isolates are present in lesions are now becoming available. For example, Cepheid has a SSTI kit that can detect S aureus and MRSA, with a reported sensitivity of 97% for MRSA in wound specimens.[75] An initial study of an immunochromatographic test for PVL that can be used with clinical specimens found the assay to have a sensitivity of 79% and specificity of 100% compared with polymerase chain reaction detection of pvl genes in the same S aureus isolates.[76] Despite these promising advances, there are currently no clinical trials to demonstrate that directing therapy against the PVL toxin improves outcome in cases of SSTI. Furthermore, the kits can be prohibitively expensive. Therefore, at this stage, such rapid diagnostics are unlikely to enter widespread clinical use, especially in the developing world.

TREATMENT OF UNCOMPLICATED SSTI CAUSED BY CA-MRSA

An important initial step in the management of staphylococcal SSTI is to recognize severe and/or complicated infection (including sepsis, toxic shock, pneumonia, and osteomyelitis). In addition, identifying certain factors that predispose to severe infection, such as extremes of age, comorbid illness (such as diabetes), malnutrition, and immunocompromised states is important. Careful clinical assessment to identify signs that suggest deeper infection or sepsis is critical. A simple algorithm for the assessment and treatment of children in the tropics who have common tropical skin infections has been developed for incorporation into the World Health Organization (WHO) Integrated Management of Childhood Illness program (**Fig. 1** and **Table 2**).[77] This algorithm, designed to assist primary health care workers, was found to be a robust tool in a validation study and is a useful guide for deciding how to proceed with the management of SSTI in children.[77]

Drainage of Abscesses

As outlined earlier, CA-MRSA frequently causes skin abscesses. In patients with small, simple abscesses (<5 cm), incision and drainage alone is usually adequate and obviates the need for antibiotic treatment.[78] However, in select situations, it may be reasonable to add an antibiotic that is active against MRSA; for example, if there is cellulitis surrounding the abscess or if adequate clinical follow-up cannot be assured.

Topical Treatments: Disinfecting Agents

In some patients with simple localized impetigo (eg, a small single lesion), the use of simple hygiene measures such as washing with clean water (±soap) often suffices as treatment by disinfecting the lesion. In addition, a variety of topical disinfecting treatments are available including hexachlorophene, chlorhexidine gluconate, povidone-iodine, and gentian violet; however, few data support their use.[79] Extensive clinical experience suggests that gentian violet is useful in simple and localized impetigo,[80] and some laboratory and clinical data suggest that gentian violet is effective against MRSA impetigo and colonization.[81,82] However, we recommend against its use in isolation in patients who have extensive impetigo, which is the most common clinical presentation in these tropical, developing countries.

Topical Treatments: Antimicrobial Agents

A Cochrane systematic review in 2004 concluded that topical treatment of localized impetigo with either mupirocin or fusidic acid is at least as effective as treatment with oral antibiotics.[83] These 2 topical agents were superior in studies comparing them with oral erythromycin, not the more routinely used agents such as cephalexin or (flu)cloxacillin. Also, the studies included in the Cochrane review were in patients with localized impetigo, not the widespread, often severe, lesions that are often seen in tropical settings. Furthermore, there is considerable risk of the rapid development of resistance for both these agents.[84–86] Other topical treatments, such as bacitracin, are either equivalent or inferior to both placebo and oral antibiotics.[83] For these reasons, we do not recommend the routine use of topical antimicrobials for treatment of impetigo in tropical regions.

Oral Antibiotics for Uncomplicated SSTI

In clinical trials for the treatment of impetigo, a consistent finding has been the high rate of clinical response to placebo (whether oral or topical); this suggests that a certain proportion of cases of impetigo will resolve without antibiotic treatment.[83] The decision to initiate oral antibiotic treatment of SSTI should be based on the extent of the disease (both in terms of number of lesions and the

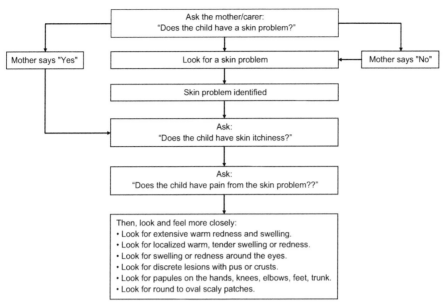

Fig. 1. Assessment algorithm for common childhood skin disorders. (*Data from* Steer AC, Tikoduadua LV, Manalac EM, et al. Validation of an integrated management of childhood illness algorithm for managing common skin conditions in Fiji. Bull World Health Organ 2009;87(3):174.)

extent of individual lesions), as well as the risk of extension of local disease and the risk of systemic bacterial invasion. In addition, there are public health considerations in trying to prevent spread to other individuals, particularly in tropical zones where poststreptococcal sequelae are common.[87] Parenteral therapy should be considered in patients with extensive disease, patients with fever, or those in whom adherence to oral therapy is likely to be poor. Intravenous therapy is indicated in patients with suspected invasive disease, as discussed later.

As outlined earlier, the most prominent pathogens that require treatment are *S pyogenes* or *S aureus*, and antibiotic choice should be directed toward both these pathogens. To date, no *S pyogenes* isolate has been found to be resistant to penicillin, and therefore a β-lactam antibiotic remains appropriate for *S pyogenes*. However, the choice of empiric antibiotic for treatment of staphylococcal SSTI is less simple and depends on local susceptibility patterns.[35] A variety of oral agents are available, including clindamycin, doxycycline, trimethoprim-sulfamethoxazole (co-trimoxazole), and linezolid. There have been no head-to-head, randomized, controlled trials of oral antibiotic therapy for CA-MRSA SSTI.

Clindamycin

In much of the United States, where the USA300 strain of CA-MRSA is most prevalent, clindamycin is commonly used for SSTI caused by CA-MRSA. Clindamycin is generally well tolerated, is well absorbed orally, with a bioavailability approaching 100%, and reaches high tissue concentrations, making it an excellent antibiotic for the treatment of soft tissue infections. Because it is a protein synthesis inhibitor, it also has the theoretic advantage of inhibiting toxin production, including PVL.[88] Its drawbacks include that it is bacteriostatic rather than bactericidal, the risk of *Clostridium difficile* infection, the need for dosing 3 to 4 times a day, poor palatability of pediatric formulations, and concerns about inducing resistance. Resistance rates to clindamycin apparently vary by strain; in the past, the USA300 strain has appeared to have been consistently susceptible to clindamycin, although recent reports suggest that this may be changing.[89,90] The situation is less clear in tropical developing regions where fewer data are available. An important caveat is the issue of inducible resistance, or macrolide-lincosamide-streptogramin B (MLSB) resistance, which is usually encoded by the *erm* gene.[91] The MLSB resistance mechanism should be tested for using the D-zone test when a staphylococcal isolate is resistant to erythromycin but susceptible to clindamycin; if the D-zone test is positive, clindamycin should not be used because of the risk of clinical failure.[92] Approximately 25% of CA-MRSA isolates in northern Australia and Hong Kong have been found to have inducible clindamycin resistance.[12,34]

Table 2
Modified WHO Integrated Management of Childhood Illness algorithm for classification of common childhood skin conditions

Sign	Diagnosis	Action
Any general danger sign (including unable to feed, vomiting all food provided, lethargy) Extensive warm redness or swelling	Very severe skin infection	Give first dose of appropriate antibiotic Refer urgently to hospital
Swelling or redness around eyes	Periorbital or orbital cellulitis	Give first dose of appropriate antibiotic Refer urgently to hospital
Localized warm tender swelling and redness	Abscess or cellulitis	Give first dose of appropriate antibiotic Refer to hospital: small abscesses (<5 cm) may be able to be drained without the need for antibiotics
Discrete sores/lesions with pus or crusts	Impetigo	If small/single impetigo lesion, consider gentian violet or simple hygiene methods such as daily cleansing with soap and clean water Otherwise, give appropriate oral antibiotic for 7 d Follow-up in 5 d
Itchiness and papules	Scabies	Provide topical permethrin skin cream Treat the whole family with permethrin cream Follow-up in 2 wk
Round to oval flat scaly patches, often itchy	Fungal infection	Give appropriate topical antifungal for 2 wk Follow-up in 2 wk
If there are not enough signs to classify in any of the above boxes OR if other signs present are not found in the above boxes	Other skin conditions	Refer to the doctor or skin clinic

Adapted from Steer AC, Tikoduadua LV, Manalac EM, et al. Validation of an integrated management of childhood illness algorithm for managing common skin conditions in Fiji. Bull World Health Organ 2009;87(3):174.

Trimethoprim-sulfamethoxazole (Co-trimoxazole)

Trimethoprim-sulfamethoxazole is also commonly used in the treatment of CA-MRSA soft tissue infection. Although it is commonly believed that *S pyogenes* is constitutively resistant to trimethoprim-sulfamethoxazole, recent data suggest that it may be effective.[93] Therefore, it may be a useful agent in tropical zones where *S pyogenes*, MSSA, and CA-MRSA are the major causes of skin infections. In a retrospective comparative study of more than 400 children with CA-MRSA SSTI, trimethoprim-sulfamethoxazole and clindamycin were found to be comparable in their effectiveness.[94] A large, randomized, controlled trial of trimethoprim-sulfamethoxazole compared with intramuscular benzathine penicillin G is currently underway in the Northern Territory of Australia (Australian and New Zealand Clinical Trials Registry ACTRN12609000858291).

Doxycycline and Linezolid

There are few data on which to base a recommendation for use of doxycycline or linezolid in the treatment of CA-MRSA SSTI. Doxycycline is inexpensive, but is contraindicated in children aged less than 8 years because of effects on dentition and bone growth. Linezolid is a protein synthesis inhibitor that has been found to be more effective than vancomycin or β-lactam antibiotics for treatment of SSTI.[95,96] However, its use is limited by its high cost and potential for side effects such as thrombocytopenia.

TREATMENT OF SEVERE INFECTIONS CAUSED BY CA-MRSA

Invasive infections with CA-MRSA have a broad spectrum of clinical presentations, with the most common being bacteremia, severe sepsis, necrotizing pneumonia, osteomyelitis, and pyomyositis. CA-MRSA–associated necrotizing fasciitis has also been reported. Vancomycin is the mainstay of treatment of these infections, although treatment failures have been reported. Many experts recommend the addition of a protein synthesis inhibitor such as clindamycin or linezolid to decrease toxin production (including PVL and the toxic shock syndrome toxin-1). In areas where clindamycin resistance is known to be high, and where linezolid is available, it may be preferable to use linezolid initially and change to a less expensive antibiotic once susceptibility results are known. Several newer agents are also available for use against CA-MRSA, although few are used in tropical developing countries; these include daptomycin, tigecycline, and quinupristin-dalfopristin.

MANAGEMENT OF COMMUNITY OUTBREAKS

Outbreaks of CA-MRSA infections have been described in sporting teams,[97] correctional facilities,[98,99] military camps,[100,101] and some small villages.[102,103] A consistent finding is the importance of personal hygiene. Infections or carriage caused by CA-MRSA have been associated with poorer hygiene practices in correctional facilities,[98] with sharing bars of soap or towels in sporting teams,[104] and using a contaminated sauna in a rural Alaskan village.[105] General recommendations provided by the Centers for Disease Control and Prevention (CDC) Web site (http://www.cdc.gov/mrsa/prevent/index.html) to prevent transmission of S aureus include covering wounds; frequent hand washing; avoiding sharing personal items; washing of soiled sheets, towels, and clothes; and regular cleaning of environmental surfaces that come into contact with the skin.

Apart from interventions aimed at improving hygiene practices, some groups have attempted more aggressive case finding and decolonization of subjects found to be colonized.[102,104,106] Such an approach terminated an outbreak of PVL positive MSSA infections in a small German village.[102] All 144 members of this village were tested for colonization by nasal swab and those who were colonized with S aureus or had current or relapsing furuncles underwent stringent decolonization procedures together with their family members. This process involved application of nasal mupirocin 3 times daily for 5 days; daily treatment of skin and hair with an octenidine-based wash solution; antiseptic treatment of the throat with 0.1% chlorhexidine solution 3 times daily; daily disinfection of personal items with an alcohol-based antimicrobial cleanser; and daily changing and washing of towels, bedclothes, and clothing. These measures eventually ended the outbreak. The ability to carry out these interventions on a village-level scale bears witness to the impressive efforts of the public health team and investigators. However, it is doubtful that this could be accomplished in other settings, particularly those with resource limitations, inadequate facilities for bathing and washing, and overcrowded households. Our experience indicates that even the basic CDC recommendations for personal hygiene are often difficult to achieve.

Casting further doubt on the efficacy of decolonizing strategies at the community level were the results of a cluster randomized, double-blind, placebo-controlled trial of targeted mupirocin therapy in CA-MRSA–colonized soldiers.[107] In this study of 3447 soldiers, there was no statistical difference in frequency of CA-MRSA infections in soldiers found to be already colonized and then given mupirocin or placebo, and no difference in incidence of SSTI or new CA-MRSA colonizations between groups of soldiers randomized to each arm. Thus, the CDC does not currently recommend routine screening for MRSA colonization, nor for eradication of colonization in infected persons or their contacts.[108]

In a community outbreak, we would suggest interventions to improve personal and community hygiene. Such strategies have been effective in halting outbreaks in a religious community[109] and in a correctional facility.[110] If an outbreak continues unabated and resources are available, then targeted screening for colonization and subsequent eradication for cases and household contacts could be considered.

VACCINATION AGAINST S AUREUS

Although there has been considerable preclinical and clinical research into both active and passive immunization against S aureus, an effective strategy has not emerged.[111] Progress in the development of a viable active vaccine has faced several hurdles, including an incomplete understanding of pathogenesis of S aureus infection.

There are few clinical and epidemiologic data to support the notion that immune protection is achieved after a single vaccination against *S aureus* infection; this is particularly the case for CA-MRSA, where recurrent SSTI is common.[24] Two vaccine candidates (StaphVAX and IsdB) have reached clinical trials.[112,113] StaphVAX is a conjugate vaccine of 2 capsular polysaccharides (CP5 and CP8) that are present in many clinical *S aureus* isolates. Two phase III trials of this vaccine have been conducted in patients on hemodialysis. The first trial was promising because it showed greater than a 50% reduction in *S aureus* bacteremia in the first 40 weeks after vaccination.[112] However, the second, larger, but as yet unpublished, trial failed to show a benefit.[111] Results of a phase II trial of a vaccine using IsdB, a cell wall protein, have similarly not been published.[111] Passive immunization using antistaphylococcal antibodies has been studied in high-risk groups, particularly premature and low birth weight infants, but clinical trials in this group have failed to show a benefit in reducing bacterial infections.[114] In summary, successful immunization against *S aureus* in high-risk groups has still not been achieved, and a routinely available antistaphylococcal vaccination for the developing world remains a more distant goal.

SUMMARY

SSTI caused by *S aureus* are very common, particularly in children, in tropical regions. The proportion of *S aureus* SSTI caused by CA-MRSA varies according to region, but is up to 25% in some areas. There are diverse CA-MRSA clones, including several that harbor PVL. Key predisposing factors for staphylococcal infections are scabies infestation, overcrowding, poor hygiene, and inadequate water supplies. In the setting of a community outbreak of staphylococcal SSTI, interventions intended to improve personal and community hygiene are likely to be the most practical, effective, and achievable. Options for oral treatment of clinical infections caused by CA-MRSA include clindamycin and trimethoprim-sulfamethoxazole. Although rapid diagnostics are now available, and 2 vaccines have reached clinical trials, neither of these is likely to be of use in tropical, developing regions in the near future.

REFERENCES

1. Skull SA, Krause V, Coombs G, et al. Investigation of a cluster of *Staphylococcus aureus* invasive infection in the top end of the Northern Territory. Aust N Z J Med 1999;29(1):66–72.
2. Andrews RM, McCarthy J, Carapetis JR, et al. Skin disorders, including pyoderma, scabies, and tinea infections. Pediatr Clin North Am 2009;56(6): 1421–40.
3. Masawe AE, Nsanzumuhire H. Scabies and other skin diseases in pre-school children in Ujamaa villages in Tanzania. Trop Geogr Med 1975;27(3): 288–94.
4. Masawe AE, Nsanzumuhire H, Mhalu F. Bacterial skin infections in preschool and school children in coastal Tanzania. Arch Dermatol 1975;111(10): 1312–6.
5. Allen AM, Taplin D. Skin infections in eastern Panama. Survey of two representative communities. Am J Trop Med Hyg 1974;23(5):950–6.
6. McDonald MI, Towers RJ, Andrews RM, et al. Low rates of streptococcal pharyngitis and high rates of pyoderma in Australian aboriginal communities where acute rheumatic fever is hyperendemic. Clin Infect Dis 2006;43(6):683–9.
7. Steer AC, Jenney AW, Kado J, et al. High burden of impetigo and scabies in a tropical country. PLoS Negl Trop Dis 2009;3(6):e467.
8. Clucas DB, Carville KS, Connors C, et al. Disease burden and health-care clinic attendances for young children in remote aboriginal communities of northern Australia. Bull World Health Organ 2008;86(4):275–81.
9. McDonald M, Dougall A, Holt D, et al. Use of a single-nucleotide polymorphism genotyping system to demonstrate the unique epidemiology of methicillin-resistant *Staphylococcus aureus* in remote aboriginal communities. J Clin Microbiol 2006;44(10):3720–7.
10. Valery PC, Wenitong M, Clements V, et al. Skin infections among indigenous Australians in an urban setting in far North Queensland. Epidemiol Infect 2008;136(8):1103–8.
11. Nagaraju U, Bhat G, Kuruvila M, et al. Methicillin-resistant *Staphylococcus aureus* in community-acquired pyoderma. Int J Dermatol 2004;43(6): 412–4.
12. Tong SY, Bishop EJ, Lilliebridge RA, et al. Community-associated strains of methicillin-resistant *Staphylococcus aureus* and methicillin-susceptible *S. aureus* in indigenous northern Australia: epidemiology and outcomes. J Infect Dis 2009;199(10): 1461–70.
13. Steer AC, Jenney AJ, Oppedisano F, et al. High burden of invasive beta-haemolytic streptococcal infections in Fiji. Epidemiol Infect 2008;136(5): 621–7.
14. Carapetis JR, Walker AM, Hibble M, et al. Clinical and epidemiological features of group a streptococcal bacteraemia in a region with hyperendemic superficial streptococcal infection. Epidemiol Infect 1999;122:59–65.

15. White AV, Hoy WE, McCredie DA. Childhood post-streptococcal glomerulonephritis as a risk factor for chronic renal disease in later life. Med J Aust 2001; 174(10):492–6.

16. McDonald M, Currie BJ, Carapetis JR. Acute rheumatic fever: a chink in the chain that links the heart to the throat? Lancet Infect Dis 2004;4:240–5.

17. Hill PC, Onyeama CO, Ikumapayi UN, et al. Bacteraemia in patients admitted to an urban hospital in West Africa. BMC Infect Dis 2007;7:2.

18. Asrat D, Amanuel YW. Prevalence and antibiotic susceptibility pattern of bacterial isolates from blood culture in Tikur Anbassa hospital, Addis Ababa, Ethiopia. Ethiop Med J 2001;39(2): 97–104.

19. Shwe TN, Nyein MM, Yi W, et al. Blood culture isolates from children admitted to medical unit III, Yangon Children's Hospital, 1998. Southeast Asian J Trop Med Public Health 2002;33(4):764–71.

20. Blomberg B, Manji KP, Urassa WK, et al. Antimicrobial resistance predicts death in Tanzanian children with bloodstream infections: a prospective cohort study. BMC Infect Dis 2007;7:43.

21. Phetsouvanh R, Phongmany S, Soukaloun D, et al. Causes of community-acquired bacteremia and patterns of antimicrobial resistance in Vientiane, Laos. Am J Trop Med Hyg 2006;75(5):978–85.

22. John R, Naraqi S, McDonnell G. The clinical spectrum of staphylococcal bacteraemia: a review of 101 Melanesian patients from Papua New Guinea. P N G Med J 1990;33(3):229–33.

23. Nickerson EK, Hongsuwan M, Limmathurotsakul D, et al. Staphylococcus aureus bacteraemia in a tropical setting: patient outcome and impact of antibiotic resistance. PLoS One 2009;4(1):e4308.

24. David MZ, Daum RS. Community-associated methicillin-resistant Staphylococcus aureus: epidemiology and clinical consequences of an emerging epidemic. Clin Microbiol Rev 2010;23(3):616–87.

25. Ghaznavi-Rad E, Nor Shamsudin M, Sekawi Z, et al. Predominance and emergence of clones of hospital-acquired methicillin-resistant Staphylococcus aureus in Malaysia. J Clin Microbiol 2010; 48(3):867–72.

26. Gadepalli R, Dhawan B, Kapil A, et al. Clinical and molecular characteristics of nosocomial methicillin-resistant Staphylococcus aureus skin and soft tissue isolates from three Indian hospitals. J Hosp Infect 2009;73(3):253–63.

27. Brown PD, Ngeno C. Antimicrobial resistance in clinical isolates of Staphylococcus aureus from hospital and community sources in southern Jamaica. Int J Infect Dis 2007;11(3):220–5.

28. Kesah C, Ben Redjeb S, Odugbemi TO, et al. Prevalence of methicillin-resistant Staphylococcus aureus in eight African hospitals and Malta. Clin Microbiol Infect 2003;9(2):153–6.

29. Lamaro-Cardoso J, de Lencastre H, Kipnis A, et al. Molecular epidemiology and risk factors for nasal carriage of Staphylococcus aureus and methicillin-resistant S. aureus in infants attending day care centers in Brazil. J Clin Microbiol 2009; 47(12):3991–7.

30. Chatterjee SS, Ray P, Aggarwal A, et al. A community-based study on nasal carriage of Staphylococcus aureus. Indian J Med Res 2009; 130(6):742–8.

31. Ribeiro J, Boyce JM, Zancanaro PQ. Prevalence of methicillin-resistant Staphylococcus aureus (MRSA) among patients visiting the emergency room at a tertiary hospital in Brazil. Braz J Infect Dis 2005; 9(1):52–5.

32. Lamaro-Cardoso J, Castanheira M, de Oliveira RM, et al. Carriage of methicillin-resistant Staphylococcus aureus in children in Brazil. Diagn Microbiol Infect Dis 2007;57(4):467–70.

33. Ruimy R, Maiga A, Armand-Lefevre L, et al. The carriage population of Staphylococcus aureus from Mali is composed of a combination of pandemic clones and the divergent Panton-Valentine leukocidin-positive genotype ST152. J Bacteriol 2008;190(11):3962–8.

34. Ho PL, Chuang SK, Choi YF, et al. Community-associated methicillin-resistant and methicillin-sensitive Staphylococcus aureus: skin and soft tissue infections in Hong Kong. Diagn Microbiol Infect Dis 2008;61(3):245–50.

35. Tong SY, McDonald MI, Holt DC, et al. Global implications of the emergence of community-associated methicillin-resistant Staphylococcus aureus in indigenous populations. Clin Infect Dis 2008; 46(12):1871–8.

36. Nubel U, Roumagnac P, Feldkamp M, et al. Frequent emergence and limited geographic dispersal of methicillin-resistant Staphylococcus aureus. Proc Natl Acad Sci U S A 2008;105(37):14130–5.

37. Liu C, Graber CJ, Karr M, et al. A population-based study of the incidence and molecular epidemiology of methicillin-resistant Staphylococcus aureus disease in San Francisco, 2004–2005. Clin Infect Dis 2008;46(11):1637–46.

38. Johnson JK, Khoie T, Shurland S, et al. Skin and soft tissue infections caused by methicillin-resistant Staphylococcus aureus USA300 clone. Emerg Infect Dis 2007;13(8):1195–200.

39. Hersh AL, Chambers HF, Maselli JH, et al. National trends in ambulatory visits and antibiotic prescribing for skin and soft-tissue infections. Arch Intern Med 2008;168(14):1585–91.

40. King MD, Humphrey BJ, Wang YF, et al. Emergence of community-acquired methicillin-resistant Staphylococcus aureus USA 300 clone as the predominant cause of skin and soft-tissue infections. Ann Intern Med 2006;144(5):309–17.

41. Moran GJ, Krishnadasan A, Gorwitz RJ, et al. Methicillin-resistant *S. aureus* infections among patients in the emergency department. N Engl J Med 2006; 355(7):666–74.

42. Chheng K, Tarquinio S, Wuthiekanun V, et al. Emergence of community-associated methicillin-resistant *Staphylococcus aureus* associated with pediatric infection in Cambodia. PLoS One 2009;4(8):e6630.

43. Fan J, Shu M, Zhang G, et al. Biogeography and virulence of *Staphylococcus aureus*. PLoS One 2009;4(7):e6216.

44. Hsu LY, Koh YL, Chlebicka NL, et al. Establishment of ST30 as the predominant clonal type among community-associated methicillin-resistant *Staphylococcus aureus* isolates in Singapore. J Clin Microbiol 2006;44(3):1090–3.

45. Tong SY, Lilliebridge RA, Bishop EJ, et al. Clinical correlates of Panton-Valentine leukocidin (PVL), PVL isoforms, and clonal complex in the *Staphylococcus aureus* population of northern Australia. J Infect Dis 2010;202(5):760–9.

46. Ng JW, Holt DC, Lilliebridge RA, et al. Phylogenetically distinct *Staphylococcus aureus* lineage prevalent among indigenous communities in northern Australia. J Clin Microbiol 2009;47(7):2295–300.

47. Estivariz CF, Park SY, Hageman JC, et al. Emergence of community-associated methicillin resistant *Staphylococcus aureus* in Hawaii, 2001–2003. J Infect 2007;54(4):349–57.

48. D'Souza N, Rodrigues C, Mehta A. Molecular characterization of methicillin-resistant *Staphylococcus aureus* with emergence of epidemic clones of sequence type (ST) 22 and ST 772 in Mumbai, India. J Clin Microbiol 2010;48(5):1806–11.

49. Breurec S, Zriouil SB, Fall C, et al. Epidemiology of methicillin-resistant *Staphylococcus aureus* lineages in five major African towns: emergence and spread of atypical clones. Clin Microbiol Infect 2010, in press. Available at: http://dx.doi.org/10.1111/j.1469-0691.2010.03219.x. Accessed September 21, 2010.

50. Enany S, Yaoita E, Yoshida Y, et al. Molecular characterization of Panton-Valentine leukocidin-positive community-acquired methicillin-resistant *Staphylococcus aureus* isolates in Egypt. Microbiol Res 2010;165(2):152–62.

51. Ghebremedhin B, Olugbosi MO, Raji AM, et al. Emergence of a community-associated methicillin-resistant *Staphylococcus aureus* strain with a unique resistance profile in southwest Nigeria. J Clin Microbiol 2009;47(9):2975–80.

52. Reyes J, Rincon S, Diaz L, et al. Dissemination of methicillin-resistant *Staphylococcus aureus* USA300 sequence type 8 lineage in Latin America. Clin Infect Dis 2009;49(12):1861–7.

53. Ho PL, Cheung C, Mak GC, et al. Molecular epidemiology and household transmission of community-associated methicillin-resistant *Staphylococcus aureus* in Hong Kong. Diagn Microbiol Infect Dis 2007;57(2):145–51.

54. Ruimy R, Armand-Lefevre L, Barbier F, et al. Comparisons between geographically diverse samples of carried *Staphylococcus aureus*. J Bacteriol 2009;191(18):5577–83.

55. Jenney A, Ritka R, Holt D, et al. Single nucleotide polymorphism genotyping of staphylococcal isolates from Fiji. In: Programs and abstracts of the Annual Scientific Meeting of the Australasian Society of Infectious Diseases. Darwin (Australia), May 26–29, 2010.

56. Chambers HF, Deleo FR. Waves of resistance: *Staphylococcus aureus* in the antibiotic era. Nat Rev Microbiol 2009;7(9):629–41.

57. Gillet Y, Issartel B, Vanhems P, et al. Association between *Staphylococcus aureus* strains carrying gene for Panton-Valentine leukocidin and highly lethal necrotising pneumonia in young immunocompetent patients. Lancet 2002;359(9308):753–9.

58. Lina G, Piemont Y, Godail-Gamot F, et al. Involvement of Panton-Valentine leukocidin-producing *Staphylococcus aureus* in primary skin infections and pneumonia. Clin Infect Dis 1999;29(5): 1128–32.

59. Bae IG, Tonthat GT, Stryjewski ME, et al. Presence of genes encoding the Panton-Valentine leukocidin exotoxin is not the primary determinant of outcome in patients with complicated skin and skin structure infections due to methicillin-resistant *Staphylococcus aureus*: results of a multinational trial. J Clin Microbiol 2009;47(12):3952–7.

60. Nickerson EK, Wuthiekanun V, Wongsuvan G, et al. Factors predicting and reducing mortality in patients with invasive *Staphylococcus aureus* disease in a developing country. PLoS One 2009; 4(8):e6512.

61. Bubeck Wardenburg J, Palazzolo-Ballance AM, Otto M, et al. Panton-Valentine leukocidin is not a virulence determinant in murine models of community-associated methicillin-resistant *Staphylococcus aureus* disease. J Infect Dis 2008;198(8): 1166–70.

62. Brown EL, Dumitrescu O, Thomas D, et al. The Panton-Valentine leukocidin vaccine protects mice against lung and skin infections caused by *Staphylococcus aureus* USA300. Clin Microbiol Infect 2009;15(2):156–64.

63. Tseng CW, Kyme P, Low J, et al. *Staphylococcus aureus* Panton-Valentine leukocidin contributes to inflammation and muscle tissue injury. PLoS One 2009;4(7):e6387.

64. Munckhof WJ, Nimmo GR, Carney J, et al. Methicillin-susceptible, non-multiresistant methicillin-resistant and multiresistant methicillin-resistant *Staphylococcus aureus* infections: a clinical, epidemiological and microbiological comparative

study. Eur J Clin Microbiol Infect Dis 2008;27(5): 355–64.

65. Muttaiyah S, Coombs G, Pandey S, et al. Incidence, risk factors and outcome of Panton-Valentine leukocidin positive methicillin-susceptible *Staphylococcus aureus* infections in Auckland, New Zealand. J Clin Microbiol 2010;48(10):3470–4.

66. Breurec S, Fall C, Pouillot R, et al. Epidemiology of methicillin-susceptible *Staphylococcus aureus* lineages in five major African towns: high prevalence of Panton-Valentine leukocidin genes. Clin Microbiol Infect 2010, in press. Available at: http://dx.doi.org/10.1111/j.1469-0691.2010.03320. x. Accessed September 21, 2010.

67. Lawrence G, Leafasia J, Sheridan J, et al. Control of scabies, skin sores and haematuria in children in the Solomon Islands: another role for ivermectin. Bull World Health Organ 2005;83(1):34–42.

68. Taplin D, Porcelain SL, Meinking TL, et al. Community control of scabies: a model based on use of permethrin cream. Lancet 1991;337:1016–8.

69. Carapetis JR, Connors C, Yarmirr D, et al. Success of a scabies control program in an Australian aboriginal community. Pediatr Infect Dis J 1997; 16(5):494–9.

70. Mahe A, Prual A, Konate M, et al. Skin diseases of children in Mali: a public health problem. Trans R Soc Trop Med Hyg 1995;89(5):467–70.

71. Ferrieri P, Dajani AS, Wannamaker LW, et al. Natural history of impetigo. I. Site sequence of acquisition and familial patterns of spread of cutaneous streptococci. J Clin Invest 1972;51(11):2851–62.

72. Hegazy AA, Darwish NM, Abdel-Hamid IA, et al. Epidemiology and control of scabies in an Egyptian village. Int J Dermatol 1999;38(4):291–5.

73. Luby SP, Agboatwalla M, Feikin DR, et al. Effect of handwashing on child health: a randomised controlled trial. Lancet 2005;366(9481):225–33.

74. Lehmann D, Tennant MT, Silva DT, et al. Benefits of swimming pools in two remote aboriginal communities in western Australia: intervention study. BMJ 2003;327(7412):415–9.

75. Wolk DM, Struelens MJ, Pancholi P, et al. Rapid detection of *Staphylococcus aureus* and methicillin-resistant *S. aureus* (MRSA) in wound specimens and blood cultures: multicenter preclinical evaluation of the Cepheid Xpert MRSA/SA skin and soft tissue and blood culture assays. J Clin Microbiol 2009;47(3):823–6.

76. Badiou C, Dumitrescu O, George N, et al. Rapid detection of *Staphylococcus aureus* Panton-Valentine leukocidin in clinical specimens by enzyme-linked immunosorbent assay and immunochromatographic tests. J Clin Microbiol 2010;48(4): 1384–90.

77. Steer AC, Tikoduadua LV, Manalac EM, et al. Validation of an integrated management of childhood illness algorithm for managing common skin conditions in Fiji. Bull World Health Organ 2009; 87(3):173–9.

78. Lee MC, Rios AM, Aten MF, et al. Management and outcome of children with skin and soft tissue abscesses caused by community-acquired methicillin-resistant *Staphylococcus aureus*. Pediatr Infect Dis J 2004;23(2):123–7.

79. Haley CE, Marling-Cason M, Smith JW, et al. Bactericidal activity of antiseptics against methicillin-resistant *Staphylococcus aureus*. J Clin Microbiol 1985;21(6):991–2.

80. MacDonald RS. Treatment of impetigo: paint it blue. BMJ 2004;329(7472):979.

81. Okano M, Noguchi S, Tabata K, et al. Topical gentian violet for cutaneous infection and nasal carriage with MRSA. Int J Dermatol 2000; 39(12):942–4.

82. Saji M, Taguchi S, Uchiyama K, et al. Efficacy of gentian violet in the eradication of methicillin-resistant *Staphylococcus aureus* from skin lesions. J Hosp Infect 1995;31(3):225–8.

83. Koning S, Verhagen AP, van Suijlekom-Smit LW, et al. Interventions for impetigo. Cochrane Database Syst Rev 2004;2:CD003261.

84. Jones JC, Rogers TJ, Brookmeyer P, et al. Mupirocin resistance in patients colonized with methicillin-resistant *Staphylococcus aureus* in a surgical intensive care unit. Clin Infect Dis 2007;45(5):541–7.

85. Alsterholm M, Flytstrom I, Bergbrant IM, et al. Fusidic acid-resistant *Staphylococcus aureus* in impetigo contagiosa and secondarily infected atopic dermatitis. Acta Derm Venereol 2010; 90(1):52–7.

86. Dobie D, Gray J. Fusidic acid resistance in *Staphylococcus aureus*. Arch Dis Child 2004; 89(1):74–7.

87. Ahn SY, Ingulli E. Acute poststreptococcal glomerulonephritis: an update. Curr Opin Pediatr 2008; 20(2):157–62.

88. Dumitrescu O, Badiou C, Bes M, et al. Effect of antibiotics, alone and in combination, on Panton-Valentine leukocidin production by a *Staphylococcus aureus* reference strain. Clin Microbiol Infect 2008;14(4):384–8.

89. Szczesiul JM, Shermock KM, Murtaza UI, et al. No decrease in clindamycin susceptibility despite increased use of clindamycin for pediatric community-associated methicillin-resistant *Staphylococcus aureus* skin infections. Pediatr Infect Dis J 2007;26(9):852–4.

90. Han LL, McDougal LK, Gorwitz RJ, et al. High frequencies of clindamycin and tetracycline resistance in methicillin-resistant *Staphylococcus aureus* pulsed-field type USA300 isolates collected at a Boston Ambulatory Health Center. J Clin Microbiol 2007;45(4):1350–2.

91. Fiebelkorn KR, Crawford SA, McElmeel ML, et al. Practical disk diffusion method for detection of inducible clindamycin resistance in *Staphylococcus aureus* and coagulase-negative staphylococci. J Clin Microbiol 2003;41(10):4740–4.

92. Siberry GK, Tekle T, Carroll K, et al. Failure of clindamycin treatment of methicillin-resistant *Staphylococcus aureus* expressing inducible clindamycin resistance in vitro. Clin Infect Dis 2003;37(9):1257–60.

93. Tong SY, Andrews RM, Kearns T, et al. Trimethoprim-sulfamethoxazole compared with benzathine penicillin for treatment of impetigo in aboriginal children: a pilot randomised controlled trial. J Paediatr Child Health 2010;46(3):131–3.

94. Hyun DY, Mason EO, Forbes A, et al. Trimethoprim-sulfamethoxazole or clindamycin for treatment of community-acquired methicillin-resistant *Staphylococcus aureus* skin and soft tissue infections. Pediatr Infect Dis J 2009;28(1):57–9.

95. Falagas ME, Siempos II, Vardakas KZ. Linezolid versus glycopeptide or beta-lactam for treatment of gram-positive bacterial infections: meta-analysis of randomised controlled trials. Lancet Infect Dis 2008;8(1):53–66.

96. Beibei L, Yun C, Mengli C, et al. Linezolid versus vancomycin for the treatment of gram-positive bacterial infections: meta-analysis of randomised controlled trials. Int J Antimicrob Agents 2010;35(1):3–12.

97. Cohen PR. The skin in the gym: a comprehensive review of the cutaneous manifestations of community-acquired methicillin-resistant *Staphylococcus aureus* infection in athletes. Clin Dermatol 2008;26(1):16–26.

98. Turabelidze G, Lin M, Wolkoff B, et al. Personal hygiene and methicillin-resistant *Staphylococcus aureus* infection. Emerg Infect Dis 2006;12(3):422–7.

99. Centers for Disease Control and Prevention. Methicillin-resistant *Staphylococcus aureus* infections in correctional facilities—Georgia, California, and Texas, 2001-2003. MMWR Morb Mortal Wkly Rep 2003;52(41):992–6.

100. Ellis MW, Hospenthal DR, Dooley DP, et al. Natural history of community-acquired methicillin-resistant *Staphylococcus aureus* colonization and infection in soldiers. Clin Infect Dis 2004;39(7):971–9.

101. Campbell KM, Vaughn AF, Russell KL, et al. Risk factors for community-associated methicillin-resistant *Staphylococcus aureus* infections in an outbreak of disease among military trainees in San Diego, California, in 2002. J Clin Microbiol 2004;42(9):4050–3.

102. Wiese-Posselt M, Heuck D, Draeger A, et al. Successful termination of a furunculosis outbreak due to lukS-lukF-positive, methicillin-susceptible *Staphylococcus aureus* in a German village by stringent decolonization, 2002–2005. Clin Infect Dis 2007;44(11):e88–95.

103. Stevens AM, Hennessy T, Baggett HC, et al. Methicillin-resistant *Staphylococcus aureus* carriage and risk factors for skin infections, southwestern Alaska, USA. Emerg Infect Dis 2010;16(5):797–803.

104. Nguyen DM, Mascola L, Brancoft E. Recurring methicillin-resistant *Staphylococcus aureus* infections in a football team. Emerg Infect Dis 2005;11(4):526–32.

105. Baggett HC, Hennessy TW, Rudolph K, et al. Community-onset methicillin-resistant *Staphylococcus aureus* associated with antibiotic use and the cytotoxin Panton-Valentine leukocidin during a furunculosis outbreak in rural Alaska. J Infect Dis 2004;189(9):1565–73.

106. Romano R, Lu D, Holtom P. Outbreak of community-acquired methicillin-resistant *Staphylococcus aureus* skin infections among a collegiate football team. J Athl Train 2006;41(2):141–5.

107. Ellis MW, Griffith ME, Dooley DP, et al. Targeted intranasal mupirocin to prevent colonization and infection by community-associated methicillin-resistant *Staphylococcus aureus* strains in soldiers: a cluster randomized controlled trial. Antimicrob Agents Chemother 2007;51(10):3591–8.

108. Gorwitz RJ, Jernigan DB, Powers JH, et al. Strategies for the clinical management of MRSA in the community: summary of an experts' meeting convened by the Centers for Disease Control and Prevention 2006. Available at: http://www.cdc.gov/ncidod/dhqp/pdf/ar/CAMRSA_ExpMtgStrategies.pdf. Accessed July 10, 2010.

109. Coronado F, Nicholas JA, Wallace BJ, et al. Community-associated methicillin-resistant *Staphylococcus aureus* skin infections in a religious community. Epidemiol Infect 2007;135(3):492–501.

110. Wootton SH, Arnold K, Hill HA, et al. Intervention to reduce the incidence of methicillin-resistant *Staphylococcus aureus* skin infections in a correctional facility in Georgia. Infect Control Hosp Epidemiol 2004;25(5):402–7.

111. Schaffer AC, Lee JC. Vaccination and passive immunisation against *Staphylococcus aureus*. Int J Antimicrob Agents 2008;32(Suppl 1):S71–8.

112. Shinefield H, Black S, Fattom A, et al. Use of a *Staphylococcus aureus* conjugate vaccine in patients receiving hemodialysis. N Engl J Med 2002;346(7):491–6.

113. Etz H, Minh DB, Henics T, et al. Identification of in vivo expressed vaccine candidate antigens from *Staphylococcus aureus*. Proc Natl Acad Sci U S A 2002;99(10):6573–8.

114. Shah PS, Kaufman DA. Antistaphylococcal immunoglobulins to prevent staphylococcal infection in very low birth weight infants. Cochrane Database Syst Rev 2009;2:CD006449.

Mosquito-Borne Hemorrhagic Fevers

Omar Lupi, MD, PhD[a,b,c],*

KEYWORDS

- Dengue • Yellow fever • Viral hemorrhagic fevers
- Mosquito-borne hemorrhagic fevers

Arbovirus is short for arthropod-borne virus. Arboviruses are a large group of viruses that are spread by invertebrate animals (arthropods), most often by biting flies (such as mosquitoes) or ticks.[1] Birds are often the reservoir of infection for mosquitoes, which can then transmit the infection to horses, other mammals, and humans that are not an essential part of the life cycle for most arboviruses (**Table 1**). This article only discusses the mosquito-borne hemorrhagic fevers in this article.

DENGUE FEVER

At the present time, dengue is considered the most important viral infection transmitted by an arthropod vector in the world terms of morbidity and mortality.[1,2] Dengue is the most severe and prevalent disease caused by flavivirus transmitted by insects. The incidence of dengue worldwide has increased dramatically in recent decades.[3] At the present, the disease is endemic in more than 100 countries in the Americas, Africa, southeast Asia, the western Pacific, and the eastern Mediterranean. With global climate change, additional countries, such as Australia may soon have endemic dengue. More than 40% of the population of the world (2.5 billion of people) is at risk for the disease.[2]

The estimate incidence of cases of dengue fever (DF) in the world is 50 to 100 million cases annually.[3,4] Between 100 to 200 suspected cases of dengue are introduced in the United States by travelers each year.[5] At present, the evolution of the disease in the Americas is similar to southeast Asia during the 1950s and 1960s.[1,2] The mortality rate of DF is less than 1%. The estimated cases of dengue hemorrhagic fever (DHF) are also high (several hundred thousand cases per year). The fatality rate of DHF is approximately 5%.[2–4,6] When patients develop dengue shock syndrome, the mortality rate can be as high as 40%. At the present, dengue is considered the most important viral infection transmitted by an arthropod vector in terms of mortality and morbidity.[2–4,6]

In order for a dengue epidemic to occur, it is necessary to have the viral pathogen, a competent vector, and a high number of susceptible human hosts. The outbreaks can have a gradual or explosive onset, depending on the strain and serotype of the dengue virus, the number of susceptible people in the population, the amount of contact between the vector and people, the population density of the vector, and the efficiency by which the vector acquires the virus.[1,2] In the United States, the *Aedes aegypti*, the main vector, is seasonably abundant in some southern states including Arizona, New Mexico, Texas, Louisiana, Mississippi, Alabama, Georgia, and parts of Florida. In addition, *A aegypti* is sporadically reported from elsewhere in the southeast and along the Atlantic seaboard (eg, North Carolina, Tennessee, South Carolina, Arkansas, New Jersey, and Maryland). Isolated dengue outbreaks have occurred in the continental United States, and sustained dengue transmission appears to be established in southern Florida.[4,6–8]

Individuals of all ages can be affected. However, elderly individuals are more likely to be at risk

Disclosures: I have no disclosures to make.
[a] Dermatology Department, Federal University of the State of Rio de Janeiro (UNI-RIO), Brazil
[b] Dermatology Department, Policlínica Geral do Rio de Janeiro, Brazil
[c] Immunology Department, Federal University of Rio de Janeiro (UFRJ), Rio de Janeiro, Brazil
* Corresponding author. Rua Frei Leandro, 16/501 - Lagoa, Zip Code 22.470-210, Rio de Janeiro/RJ, Brazil.
E-mail address: omarlupi@globo.com

Dermatol Clin 29 (2011) 33–38
doi:10.1016/j.det.2010.09.009

Table 1
Mosquito-borne infections related to arboviruses

Bunyaviridae	Arbovirus encephalitis: La Crosse encephalitis, California encephalitis Rift Valley fever[b]
Flaviviridae	Arbovirus encephalitis: Japanese encephalitis, Australian encephalitis, St Louis encephalitis, West Nile fever[a] Dengue fever,[b] Yellow fever,[b] Zika fever[a]
Togaviridae	Arbovirus encephalitis: eastern equine encephalomyelitis, western equine encephalomyelitis, Venezuelan equine encephalomyelitis Chikungunya[a] O'Nyong-nyong fever,[a] Ross River fever[a]

[a] With skin or mucosal lesions.
[b] Hemorrhagic manifestations.

because of coexisting medical conditions. Ninety percent of patients with DHF are younger than 15 years. All races can be affected by the disease.[4,5]

DF can be caused by any of the four serotypes of dengue virus: DEN-1, DEN-2, DEN-3, and DEN-4. After a bout of dengue caused by any particular serotypye, people acquire immunity to that serotype. They can, however, be infected by any (or all) of the other three serotypes, and each successive infection may have more dire clinical consequences.[3,4] The only vertebrate hosts of the dengue virus are people. There is a jungle cycle between arthropod vectors and monkeys that plays no role in human disease.

Clinical Presentation

People with dengue can have a spectrum of clinical illness ranging from a nonspecific viral syndrome to severe and fatal hemorrhagic disease. The dengue virus infection can lead to one of the four different consequences: classical dengue, hemorrhagic dengue, dengue shock syndrome, asymptomatic infection, and less common manifestations such as hepatitis.[7]

Classical dengue, also called DF, is characterized by fever, headache, myalgia, and rash. DHF is a separate clinical entity and consists in a more virulent form of dengue virus infection.[7] In the past, dengue used to be called breakbone,

fever because the disease sometimes cause severe joint and muscle pain that feels like bones are breaking.[7]

Mild hemorrhagic symptoms (including gingival bleeding, petechiae, and a positive tourniquet test) can be seen in approximately one-third of the patients with classical dengue.[1,3,7]

Classical dengue

The most frequent form of disease is when the host has primary infection with classical dengue. Abrupt fever is the initial manifestation and can be associated or followed by headache, severe myalgia, retro-orbital pain, anorexia, vomiting, nausea, arthralgia, and fatigue. In 3 to 4 days, a morbilliform eruption (**Fig. 1**) or a scarlatiniform rash can appear.[7] This rash is centrifugal, and it is common to detect palmo-plantar edema associated with pruritus (**Fig. 2**). In children, abdominal pain is more frequent. The headache of classical dengue occurs predominantly in the frontal region and can be the chief complaint because of its intensity.[1,5] Although the rash is usually composed of macules and slightly elevated papules, it can also be purely macular or even urticarial; such cases are not easy to differentiate from a benign drug eruption, perhaps even to those medications used to control the symptoms.

Patients with classical dengue also can have lymphadenopathy and tender hepatomegaly. Hemorrhagic manifestations are not exclusively seen in DHF and also can be observed in classical dengue (**Fig. 3**).

DHF

The most important risk factors for this form are[2–4,6,7]

A history of another episode of dengue in the past (preferably a confirmed episode)

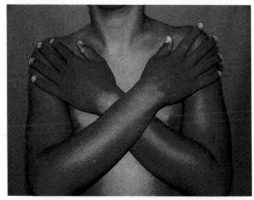

Fig. 1. Morbilliform eruption of dengue fever.

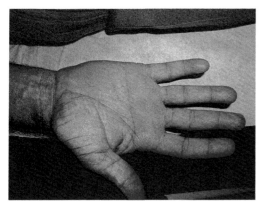

Fig. 2. Palmar edema and erythema in dengue fever.

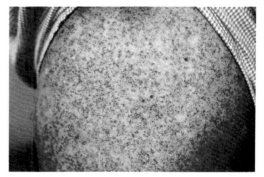

Fig. 4. Diseminated petecchiae in dengue hemorrhagic fever.

Lactating infants born from mothers who had dengue

Children younger than 12 years of age (in the southeast of Asia)

Females

When the serotype DEN-2 causes the second infection

Caucasians.

In DHF, the fever also starts abruptly, similar to classical dengue; however in days 3 to 8 of the disease evolution, characteristic findings of DHF appear (**Fig. 4**). In this period, evidence of plasma leakage in addition to bleeding and low platelets levels in the blood can be observed.[2]

The hemodynamic and systemic changes caused by the increase in the vascular permeability lead to a relative hypovolemia (eventually shock), interstitial edema, and serosal effusion.[3,4] The hemorrhagic manifestations of DHF are more severe than in the classical dengue. The patients with DHF can have moderate-to-severe thrombocytopenia and coagulation disturbances. The lethality ranges from 5% to 50% and averages 12%.[7] Recovery is observed in most of the patients.

The initial clinical picture of DHF is similar to the initial presentation of classical dengue. Hemorrhagic manifestations (such as cutaneous ecchymoses and petechiae, hematemesis, melena, hemoptysis, and subconjunctival hemorrhage) and cavitary effusions (such as ascites or pleural effusions) can be observed from the second or third day of the disease on.[7] However, hemorrhagic manifestations are not always seen in the course of DHF. The tourniquet test usually gives a positive result in DHF.[7]

Diagnosis

Clinical history includes

Recent travel to an area where dengue is endemic

Initial symptoms that include sudden onset of high fever (temperature >101° F), chills, and a severe ache of the head, back, and extremities

Dengue shock syndrome, which can be seen after dengue hemorrhagic syndrome, with symptoms of respiratory and circulatory failure that is often fatal

Uncommonly, diarrhea.

Physical examination should include

Hemorrhagic manifestations as epistaxis, purpura, petechiae and ecchymosis, which can occur in patients with DHF

The tourniquet test, which can be positive in more than 50% of the cases.

Complementary tests

Many serologic tests have been used for the diagnosis of dengue, which will detect any of the four serotypes but do not reliably distinguish among the four. Examples include immunoglobulin M (IgM) capture enzyme linked immunosorbent assay (MAC-ELISA), indirect IgG ELISA, complement

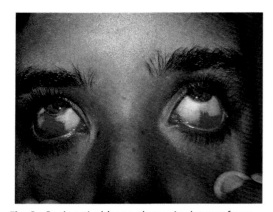

Fig. 3. Conjunctival hemorrhages in dengue fever.

fixation (CF), hemagglutination–inhibition and neutralization test. The high cross-reactivity observed with these tests is considered a limitation of these techniques. Some commonly used methods for viral isolation are: inoculation on mosquito cell cultures, inoculation on mammalian cell cultures, intrathoracic inoculation of adult mosquitoes, and intracerebral inoculation of newborn mice. Some useful new diagnostic techniques that have been developed are: reverse transcriptase–polymerase chain reaction (RT-PCR) and nucleic acid hybridization.[3,4,6]

ELISA is a commonly used technique for the diagnosis of dengue by serology. RT-PCR is a very important test, because it can detect dengue viruses up to the 10th day after the onset of the symptoms. However, ELISA does not identify the dengue virus serotype causing the current infection, thus molecular techniques will possibly have a very important role in the diagnosis of dengue in the near future.[4] At the present, the diagnosis of dengue is based on viral isolation, serology, and RNA detection.

Treatment and Prevention

The treatment of dengue is supportive and nonspecific. Hydration is a very important component of the therapy for dengue. Besides fluid replacement, patients can also benefit from bed rest and the use of analgesics and antipyretics.[7] Patients with hypotension or in disseminated intravascular coagulation (DIC) need to be admitted to the intensive care unit.

Most patients with dengue recover spontaneously after 1 week from the beginning of the appropriate therapy. In the cases of classical dengue or uncomplicated hemorrhagic dengue, patients can be discharged after 2 days without fever. The average time that the patients stay away from work is 10 days from the onset; however fatigue can continue through a prolonged convalescence period.[7]

The mortality of DHF may be reduced to less than 1% with adequate intensive supportive therapy. The main feature of DHF clinical management is the maintenance of an adequate circulating fluid volume. The use of high doses of corticosteroids has not been shown to change the mortality rates in the case of severe bleeding and shock syndrome.[7]

Acetaminophen (paracetamol) is the drug of choice for the treatment of fever and pain. Aspirin and nonsteroidal anti-inflammatory drugs (NSAIDs) are contraindicated, since they are associated with the increase risk of hemorrhagic manifestations. At present, there is no specific antiviral drug to treat dengue infections.[7]

There are no dengue vaccines available yet. Mosquito control programs against sylvatic infections are not cost-effective. For the urban cycle, elimination of mosquito breeding sites and organophosphate spraying are beneficial but must be continuously supported.

YELLOW FEVER

The name yellow fever (YF) comes from the dramatic and intense jaundice that occurs in severe cases of this disease. It is caused by the yellow fever virus, the prototypic virus of the family *Flaviviridae*. This is a mosquito-borne hemorrhagic fever that causes severe hepatic injury and often death, and it was once one of the great scourges of the world. YF's clinical course involves two distinct phases that are separated by a transient remission. The first phase has viremia, and the second involves multiorgan dysfunction and hemorrhage of varying degree. In spite of an effective vaccine, YF remains a major public health problem in equatorial Africa and the jungles of South America.[9]

The World Health Organization (WHO) estimates 200,000 cases annually with 30,000 deaths, although significant under-reporting and misidentification can occur. Before the 1900s, there were also outbreaks in Europe, the Caribbean, and Central America and North America. YF has never been reported in Asia, although WHO considers the area to be at risk, because the appropriate vectors and suitable primate hosts exist there. Nine South American countries have endemic YF, with Bolivia, Brazil, Ecuador, Columbia, and Peru considered the highest risk.[9] Peak transmission in South America occurs via sylvatic cycle from monkey hosts mostly to young men, from January to March when peak rainfall and humidity coincide with forest-clearing activities. Incidence in Africa occurs during the late rainy season, with background immunity the primary factor in determining age distribution. African countries in which YF is endemic include Atlantic coastal countries from Angola to Guinea, as well as Sudan.[9,10]

There are four topotypes (geographic genetic types): two in Africa (one occurring in the eastern countries and the other occurring in the western countries), and two in South America (only one of which has been identified as causing outbreaks).[9,10] The virus primarily affects people and primates. Transmission can be horizontal by the biting mosquito as the vector between one animal and another, or vertical (transovarial from infected female mosquitoes to their progeny). The mosquito vectors include members of the culicine genus, *Aedes,* or, in South America, members of the closely related genus, *Haemagogus*. There are three cycles of YF: sylvatic, urban, and intermediate. In sylvatic YF, the life cycle is involves monkeys and mosquitoes (eg, an infected monkey is bitten by a wild mosquito, which then is able to transmit the virus to uninfected monkeys). Sporadic human cases occur when infected sylvatic mosquitoes transmit from the virus to someone working or traveling through the jungle, usually a tropical rainforest.

Urban YF is transmitted directly from human to human via an infective domestic mosquito. This lifecycle requires only people, not sylvatic monkey reservoirs, and large outbreaks and epidemics occur. Intermediate YF involves transmission from a semidomestic mosquito to both monkeys and people. This mode occurs in the zone of emergence in the African savannah, which borders equatorial forests and has high concentrations of vectors and monkeys.[9] Intermediate YF may produce smaller outbreaks.

After inoculation, the virus replicates in regional lymph nodes, followed by dissemination through the bloodstream to other tissues, such as bone marrow, myocardium, liver, and spleen. In the liver, the virus infects Kupffer cells and then certain hepatocytes, leading to coagulative necrosis. The bleeding diathesis that occurs with YF is a result of depletion of hepatic clotting factors, platelet dysfunction, and intravascular coagulation.

Clinical Manifestations

The spectrum of disease with YF ranges from a nonspecific febrile illness to a fulminating, sometimes fatal illness. The characteristic course of disease progresses through three phases, known as the periods of infection, remission, and intoxication. Patients with YF infection may demonstrate the Faget sign, which is high fever with a paradoxically slow pulse (brdaycardia). The most significant integumentary manifestations, other than profound jaundice of the skin and sclerae, are the petechiae and ecchymosis associated with the bleeding diathesis. This is likely due to decreased hepatic synthesis of vitamin K-dependent factors as well as increased vascular permeability, altered platelet function, and ultimately disseminated intravascular coagulopathy.[9]

During the phase of intoxication, renal manifestations may include albuminuria and delerium, seizures, and coma. The jaundice associated with YF may not be significant and may be clinically undetectable until detected on postmortem examination. Signs that often precede death include worsening jaundice, hemorrhage, hypotension, oliguria, azotemia, and rising pulse. Poor prognostic indicators include hypothermia, hypoglycemia, intractable hiccups, agitation, delerium, stupor, and coma. Rarely, late death during convalescence occurs owing to cardiac or renal involvement.

Diagnosis

Laboratory findings are nonspecific and include leukopenia, elevated bilirubin and transaminases, albuminuria, thrombocytopenia, and prolonged prothrombin and bleeding time. Transaminases remain elevated for at least 2 months. An electrocardiogram may show nonspecific ST changes.

The YF virus can be isolated most easily during the earliest days of disease; however, serum up to 2 weeks after disease onset and postmortem hepatic tissue also can be used. Antibodies can be detected by hemagglutination inhibition (HI), CF and immunofluorescent assay (IFA) tests, indirect immunofluorescence, ELISA, and radioimmunoassay (RIA). Clinical suspicion must be high in patients from endemic or epidemic areas or with recent travel history. Specific IgM or a rise in antibody titer in paired serum samples is diagnostic. Serologic cross-reaction does occur with other flaviviruses.[9,10]

Treatment and Prevention

The mainstay of treatment continues to be supportive care. Antiviral therapies are not effective against this virus, and no specific therapy is available. The most important factor for prevention is immunization with a live attenuated strain of YF virus. This is recommended at least 7 to 10 days before traveling to endemic areas. Seroconversion occurs in 95% of vaccine recipients within 1 week. Although the vaccine is recommended every 10 years, immunity may be lifelong. Serious adverse effects from the vaccine are rare. The vaccine is not recommended for children under 6 months of age, pregnant women (except during an emergency vaccination campaign), persons with allergy to egg products, and persons with immunodeficiency or taking immunosuppressive medications.[9,10]

The Pan American Health Organization had vector control programs in the 1950s and 1960s that virtually eliminated *Ae. aegypti* in most countries. However, the programs were not continued, and reinfestation has occurred in all Latin American countries except Chile and Uruguay.[9,10] Mosquito control programs against sylvatic infections are not cost-effective. For the urban cycle, elimination of mosquito breeding sites, treatment of potable water, and organophosphate spraying are beneficial but must be continuously supported.

The United States has *Ae. aegypti* vector present in the southeastern region, and is therefore a potential area of epidemic in the future.

REFERENCES

1. Lupi O, Tyring SK. Tropical dermatology: viral tropical diseases. J Am Acad Dermatol 2003;49:979–1000 [quiz: 1000–2].
2. Lupi O, Spinelli L. Dengue. In: Tyring S, Lupi O, Hengge U, editors. Tropical dermatology. Oxford (UK): Elsevier; 2005. p. 136–41.
3. Centers for Disease Control and Prevention. Division of vector-bourne infectious diseases. Available at: http://www.cdc.gov/ncidod/dvbid/dengue/index.htm. Accessed September 1, 2010.
4. Halstead SB. Dengue. Curr Opin Infect Dis 2002;15:461–6.
5. Centers for Disease Control and Prevention (CDC). Travel-associated Dengue surveillance - United States, 2006–2008. MMWR Morb Mortal Wkly Rep 2010;59(23):715–9. Available at: http://www.cdc.gov/mmwr/preview/mmwrhtml/mm5923a3.htm. Accessed September 1, 2010.
6. Guzmán MG, Kourí G. Dengue: an update. Lancet Infect Dis 2002;2:33–42.
7. Lupi O, Carneiro CG, Castelo Branco I. Manifestações mucocutâneas da dengue. [Mucocutaneous Manifestations of Dengue]. An Bras Dermatol 2007;82(4):291–305 [in Portuguese].
8. Centers for Disease Control and Prevention (CDC). Locally acquired Dengue—Key West, Florida, 2009–2010. MMWR Morb Mortal Wkly Rep 2010;59(19):577–81. Available at: http://www.cdc.gov/mmwr/preview/mmwrhtml/mm5919a1.htm. Accessed September 1, 2010.
9. National Center for Infectious Diseases. Summary of health information for international travel (the blue sheet). Available at: http://www.cdc.gov/travel/bluesheet.htm. Accessed February 13, 2000.
10. McFarland JM, Baddour LM, Nelson JE, et al. Imported yellow fever in a United States citizen. Clin Infect Dis 1997;25:1143–7.

Immune Reconstitution Inflammatory Syndrome and Tropical Dermatoses

Erin Huiras Amerson, MD*, Toby A. Maurer, MD

KEYWORDS

- HIV infection
- Immune reconstitution inflammatory syndrome
- Immune restoration disease • Leprosy • Leishmaniasis
- Tropical dermatology

Tropical regions, including sub-Saharan Africa, the Caribbean, Latin America, India, and Southeast Asia, account for more than 80% of human immunodeficiency (HIV) infections around the globe.[1] The intersection of the HIV pandemic and tropical infectious diseases is inevitable; however, the lack of sophisticated medical infrastructure and diagnostic techniques, along with underreporting from these regions, has limited the understanding of how the epidemiology and clinical course of tropical infections is affected by coinfection with HIV, and much of the existing literature describes cases noted in immigrants to the developed world. As access to highly active antiretroviral therapy (HAART) in tropical regions increases, so does the understanding of its effect on persons coinfected with HIV and tropical infections.

The immune reconstitution inflammatory syndrome (IRIS), also known as immune restoration disease or immune reconstitution syndrome, is a well-documented but poorly understood phenomenon. IRIS occurs in the setting of HAART-induced immune restoration and is best described as a deregulated immunologic response to a previously existing pathogen or antigen, which then causes new or worsening clinical disease. In other words, as the HIV patient's immune system improves under HAART, it reacts to existing but clinically quiescent pathogens and immunologically ignored antigens in unexpected ways. IRIS typically occurs in the initial weeks or months after starting HAART and subsequent immune reconstitution. There are 2 principal types of IRIS that occur: unmasking IRIS, in which a previously unrecognized infection becomes clinically apparent as immune reconstitution occurs, and paradoxical IRIS, which causes clinical deterioration of a previously recognized and sometimes treated infection. IRIS lacks a clear case definition, and diagnostic biomarkers have remained elusive. The only reliable predictors of IRIS risk are a low CD4$^+$ nadir and pre-existing opportunistic infection.[2–4] Shelburne and colleagues[2] proposed the following clinical criteria for IRIS: "(1) HIV infection, (2) receiving HAART, (3) decrease in HIV-1 RNA viral load, (4) increase in the level of CD4$^+$ cells from baseline, and (5) clinical symptoms consistent with an inflammatory process whose clinical course is not consistent with the expected progression of a previously diagnosed opportunistic infection, expected progression of a newly diagnosed opportunistic infection, or drug toxicity."[2(p168)] In reality, IRIS probably represents a collection of unique disorders, each with a distinct immunopathogenesis driven by the interaction of pathogen-specific immune responses and host characteristics (eg, degree of HIV-induced immunosuppression and immunodysregulation, host genetics,

Department of Dermatology, University of California, San Francisco, 1701 Divisidero Street, 3rd Floor, San Francisco, CA 94115, USA
* Corresponding author.
E-mail address: HuirasEE@derm.ucsf.edu

Dermatol Clin 29 (2011) 39–43
doi:10.1016/j.det.2010.09.007
0733-8635/11/$ – see front matter. Published by Elsevier Inc.

and possibly the inflammatory milieu created by coinfection with other pathogens).[5] IRIS may be simply a symptomatic inconvenience for a patient or may cause significant morbidity and mortality, affecting vital organs with excessive inflammation (eg, cytomegalovirus retinitis or cryptococcal meningitis). Distinguishing IRIS from opportunistic disease caused by persistent immunodeficiency, treatment failure, or adverse drug reaction presents significant diagnostic and therapeutic challenges.

The emergence of the HIV/AIDS pandemic in the tropical developing world and the subsequent rollout of HAART in these regions have led to numerous reports of IRIS occurring in association with tropical infections. The factors known to predispose to IRIS, such as very low CD4$^+$ cell count before initiation of antiretroviral therapy and preexisting opportunistic infection, are far more likely to be encountered in these regions. Although most articles focus on IRIS caused by leprosy and leishmaniasis, IRIS has also been reported with helminthic infections (eg, schistosomiasis, strongyloidiasis) and fungal infections (eg, histoplasmosis, sporotrichosis, and penicilliosis), and many of these infections have cutaneous manifestations. With the massive burden of HIV infection in the tropical world, it is reasonable to anticipate that the range of reported tropical dermatoses with associated IRIS will continue to expand.

Relatively few IRIS events have been reported in association with parasitic helminthic infections endemic to much of the tropical world. This underreporting may reflect underdiagnosis or result from the helper T cell (T_H) 2 immunologic shift caused by advancing HIV, because T_H2-type cytokines are made during an appropriate response to many parasitic infections.[6]

This article focuses on dermatoses endemic to tropical regions that have been reported to precipitate cutaneous IRIS events, including leprosy, leishmaniasis, penicilliosis, sporotrichosis, and strongyloidiasis.

LEPROSY

Early in the HIV epidemic, HIV was speculated to lead to a significant increase in the prevalence of leprosy in endemic regions.[7] Although coinfection with HIV and *Mycobacterium leprae* has been reported frequently in tropical regions, mostly in Brazil, India, and sub-Saharan Africa, the HIV epidemic does not seem to have substantially altered the epidemiology of leprosy in these regions.[8–11] HIV infection does not seem to significantly increase the risk of becoming infected with *M leprae*, and HIV coinfection does not predict a worse outcome.[12] Furthermore, coinfected individuals

experience a similar treatment response rate as HIV-negative patients with leprosy.[11]

Even in the absence of HIV infection, paradoxic reactions reminiscent of IRIS have long been observed before, during, or after multidrug therapy (MDT) for leprosy. Termed as type I reactions, a subset of individuals experience inflammation of existing leprosy lesions soon after starting antileprous therapy, usually within weeks. These reactions are thought to be caused by increased cell-mediated immunity to the lepra bacilli. When type I reactions occur after MDT, they are called reversal reactions. On occasion, type 1 reactions occur even in the absence of therapy and are thought to be caused by a shift in host cell-mediated immunity to the pathogen; these reactions are termed upgrading when the clinical picture shifts toward the paucibacillary end of the spectrum and downgrading when the clinical picture shifts toward the multibacillary pole. Type 1 reactions present clinically with a cellulitis-like inflammation of existing lesions, sometimes with ulceration or necrosis, and can cause significant morbidity because of inflammatory nerve damage. When type 1 reactions occur, they are typically treated with prednisone or other immunosuppressive agents.[13]

HIV-leprosy coinfection might be expected to increase the prevalence of multibacillary disease. Instead, HIV infection does not seem to alter the ratio of lepromatous to tuberculoid leprosy; in fact, it seems to predispose to paucibacillary rather than multibacillary disease.[11,14] Even in advanced HIV infection, the histologic features of leprosy, including granuloma formation, appear to be preserved, indicating that the local cell-mediated immune response is intact.[11]

Deps and Lockwood[15] proposed the following case definition for leprosy IRIS: (1) leprosy and/or leprosy type 1 reaction presenting within 6 months of starting HAART, (2) advanced HIV infection, (3) low CD4$^+$ cell count before starting HAART, and (4) increase in CD4$^+$ cell count after starting HAART. To date, more than 30 reported cases of IRIS associated with leprosy infection have met these criteria. Most cases presented as unmasking of previously unrecognized leprosy, of which most manifested as borderline paucibacillary disease. Several reports have included descriptions of lesions that initially presented with, or later developed, symptoms clinically consistent with type I reactions, including inflammation and ulceration or necrosis of prior typical leprosy lesions; neuritis, however, seems to be rare.[12,16–31] Talhari and colleagues[32] reported 2 individuals who had unmasking of multibacillary disease and experienced upgrading to paucibacillary disease accompanied by inflammation and ulceration of existing lesions. Paradoxical reactions, where a person with known leprosy developed reversal-like reactions within weeks to months of starting HAART, have been reported less frequently.[25,26,30,33]

Supporting the hypothesis that HAART-induced immune restoration unmasked these events, Couppié and colleagues[34] determined in French Guiana the adjusted hazard ratio for a new diagnosis of leprosy in those receiving HAART for 3 months or more over HIV-infected untreated patients was 18.5 (95% CI: 1.6-217; P = .02). Nunes Sarno and colleagues[14] also found that initiation of HAART was associated with a new diagnosis of leprosy (P = .001).

Published case reports that included outcomes consistently described clinical improvement after the initial IRIS event. In addition, patients treated with prednisone had eventual improvement of their disease without serious adverse effects.

LEISHMANIASIS

Leishmania infection in patients coinfected with HIV occurs at anywhere between 10 to 100 times the expected rate.[35] In association with HAART-induced immune restoration, 3 clinical variations of leishmaniasis with cutaneous findings have been reported: diffuse mucocutaneous leishmaniasis, post- or para−kala-azar dermal leishmaniasis (PKDL), and sporotrichoid dermal and subcutaneous nodules. Both unmasking and paradoxical reactions are reported. Diffuse mucocutaneous leishmaniasis, an unusual clinical variant of New World disease that typically occurs in anergic individuals, has been described in 3 cases in patients from Brazil and one in a Nicaraguan immigrant to the United States.[36−38] From the Old World, 7 cases of leishmanial IRIS events have been reported presenting as PKDL.[39−44] In addition, 1 case of paradoxical clinical deterioration of sporotrichoid nodules caused by *Leishmania major* was reported in a Senegalese immigrant to France.[45]

PENICILLIOSIS

Penicillium marneffei is a dimorphic environmental fungus that causes infection almost exclusively in northern Thailand and adjacent areas of Southeast Asia. Disseminated infection often presents as multiple crusted molluscum contagiosum-like papules in the skin. To date, three cases of *Penicillium marneffei* associated IRIS have been reported. Gupta and colleagues[46] reported an HIV-infected patient in India, without cutaneous disease, who developed new lymphadenopathy shortly after starting HAART; *P marneffei* was isolated from a lymph node aspirate. Saikia and colleagues[47] reported another Indian patient with HIV who developed widespread molluscum-like lesions on the face, extremities, and scrotum; culture from his skin and blood grew *P marneffei*. Saikia and colleagues[48] also reported paradoxical worsening of *P marneffei* skin lesions, along with development of fever, arthritis, and lymphadenopathy, in a 12 year old boy 1 month after starting HAART.

SPOROTRICHOSIS

A report from Brazil described 2 patients with cutaneous IRIS associated with *Sporothrix schenckii* infection. One individual had biopsy-proven, culture-positive sporotrichosis before starting HAART and initially responded to oral itraconazole. After 6 weeks on HAART, the patient experienced paradoxical deterioration with reactivation of old lesions and development of new cutaneous and mucosal lesions. The second patient had no cutaneous findings before HAART but experienced unmasking of sporotrichosis of the left hand 5 weeks into HAART; culture of lesion exudates grew *S schenckii*. Both patients recovered well with a combination of amphotericin B and itraconazole.[49]

STRONGYLOIDIASIS

One report of IRIS-associated disseminated strongyloidiasis describes an Eritrean immigrant to Italy whose infection was unmasked 2 months after initiating HAART. The patient's symptoms included itchy skin, fever, cough, vomiting, diarrhea, epigastric pain, and eosinophilia. He improved after thiabendazole treatment.[50]

SUMMARY

IRIS occurs frequently in association with some tropical infections, and clinicians who treat HIV-infected individuals from tropical regions should be aware of the possibility of IRIS after starting HAART. This awareness helps the clinician from mistakenly attributing IRIS-associated signs and symptoms to treatment failure or an adverse drug reaction. More data are needed to understand the etiopathogenesis of IRIS associated with tropical dermatoses and optimize diagnosis and treatment of IRIS symptoms.

REFERENCES

1. Available at: http://www.avert.org/worldstats.htm. Accessed August 1, 2010.

2. Shelburne SA, Montes M, Hamill RJ. Immune reconstitution inflammatory syndrome: more answers, more questions. J Antimicrob Chemother 2006; 57(2):167–70.

3. Ratnam I, Chiu C, Kandala NB, et al. Incidence and risk factors for immune reconstitution inflammatory syndrome in an ethnically diverse HIV type 1-infected cohort. Clin Infect Dis 2006;42(3):418–27.

4. French MA, Lenzo N, John M, et al. Immune restoration disease after the treatment of immunodeficient HIV-infected patients with highly active antiretroviral therapy. HIV Med 2000;1(2):107–15.

5. French MA. Immune reconstitution inflammatory syndrome: a reappraisal. Clin Infect Dis 2009;48:101–7.

6. Lawn SD, Wilkinson RJ. Immune reconstitution disease associated with parasitic infections following antiretroviral treatment. Parasite Immunol 2006;28:625–33.

7. Turk JL, Rees RJ. AIDS and leprosy. Lepr Rev 1988; 59:193–4.

8. Lucas S. Human immunodeficiency virus and leprosy. Lepr Rev 1993;64:97–103.

9. Frommel D, Teykle-Haimonot R, Verdie M, et al. HIV infection and leprosy: a four-year survey in Ethiopia. Lancet 1994;344:165–6.

10. van den Broek J, Chum HJ, Swai R, et al. Association between leprosy and HIV infection in Tanzania. Int J Lepr Other Mycobact Dis 1997;65:203–10.

11. Ustiantowski AP, Lawn SD, Lockwood DN. Interactions between HIV and leprosy: a paradox. Lancet Infect Dis 2006;6:350–60.

12. Pereira GAS, Stefani MMA, Araujo Filho JA, et al. Human immunodeficiency virus type 1 (HIV-1) and Mycobacterium leprae co-infection: HIV-1 subtypes and clinical, immunologic, and histopathologic profiles in a Brazilian cohort. Am J Trop Med Hyg 2004;71(5):679–84.

13. Britton WJ, Lockwood DN. Leprosy reactions: current and future approaches to management. Bailliere's Clin Infect Dis 1997;4:1–23.

14. Nunes Sarno E, Illarramendi X, Costa Nery JA, et al. HIV-M. leprae interaction: can HAART modify the course of leprosy? Public Health Rep 2008;123:206–12.

15. Deps PD, Lockwood DN. Leprosy occurring as immune reconstitution syndrome. Trans R Soc Trop Med Hyg 2008;102:966–8.

16. Visco-Comandini U, Longo B, Cuzzi T, et al. Tuberculoid leprosy in a patient with AIDS: a manifestation of immune restoration syndrome. Scand J Infect Dis 2004;36:881–3.

17. Narang T, Dogra S, Kaur I. Borderline tuberculoid leprosy with type 1 reaction in an HIV patient—a phenomenon of immune reconstitution. Int J Lepr Other Mycobact Dis 2005;73(3):203–5.

18. Singal A, Mehta S, Pahndhi D. Immune reconstitution inflammatory syndrome in an HIV-positive leprosy patient. Lepr Rev 2006;77:76–80.

19. Kharkar V, Bhor UH, Mahajan S, et al. Type I lepra reaction presenting as immune reconstitution inflammatory syndrome. Indian J Dermatol Venereol Leprol 2007;73:253–6.

20. Bussone G, Charlier C, Bille E, et al. Case report: unmasking leprosy: an unusual immune reconstitution inflammatory syndrome in a patient infected with human immunodeficiency virus. Am J Trop Med Hyg 2010;83(1):13–4.

21. Deps PD, Gripps CG, Madureira BPR, et al. Immune reconstitution syndrome associated with leprosy: two cases. Int J STD AIDS 2008;19:135–6.

22. Kar HK, Sharma P, Bhardwaj M. Type 1 reaction in a HIV seropositive patient, after antiretroviral therapy: an immune reconstitution inflammatory syndrome. Lepr Rev 2009;80:85–8.

23. Sharma P, Bhardwaj M, Kar HK. Inoculation leprosy and HIV co-infection: a rare case with nerve involvement preceding development of skin patch and type 1 reaction as immune reconstitution syndrome following antiretroviral therapy. Indian J Lepr 2009; 81(2):75–9.

24. Couppie P, Abel S, Voinchet H, et al. Immune reconstitution inflammatory syndrome associated with HIV and leprosy. Arch Dermatol 2004;140(8): 997–1000.

25. Batista MD, Porro AM, Maeda SM, et al. Leprosy reversal reaction as immune reconstitution inflammatory syndrome in patients with AIDS. Clin Infect Dis 2008;46:e56–60.

26. Martiniuk F, Rao SD, Rea TH, et al. Leprosy as immune reconstitution inflammatory syndrome in HIV-positive persons. Emerg Infect Dis 2007;13(9): 1438–40.

27. Talhari C, Roberto P, Machado L, et al. Shifting of the clinical spectrum of leprosy in an HIV-positive patient: a manifestation of immune reconstitution inflammatory syndrome? Lepr Rev 2007;78:151–4.

28. Lawn Wood. Lockwood borderline tuberculoid leprosy: an immune reconstitution phenomenon in a human immunodeficiency virus-infected person. Clin Infect Dis 2003;36:e5–6.

29. Pignataro P, da Silva Rocha A, Costa Nery JA, et al. Leprosy and AIDS: two cases of increasing inflammatory reactions at the start of highly active antiretroviral therapy. Eur J Clin Microbiol Infect Dis 2004;23(5):408–11.

30. Menezes VM, Sales AM, Illarramendi X, et al. Leprosy reaction as a manifestation of immune reconstitution inflammatory syndrome: a case series of a Brazilian cohort. AIDS 2009;23(5):641–3.

31. Handa S, Narang T, Wanchu A. Dermatologic immune restoration syndrome: report of five cases from a tertiary care center in north India. J Cutan Med Surg 2008;12(3):126–32.

32. Talhari C, De Lima Ferreira LC, Araujo JR, et al. Immune reconstitution inflammatory syndrome or

upgrading type 1 reaction? Report of two AIDS patients presenting a shifting from borderline lepromatous leprosy to borderline tuberculoid leprosy. Lepr Rev 2008;79:429–35.

33. Chow D, Okinaka L, Souza S, et al. Hansen's disease with HIV: a case of immune reconstitution disease. Hawaii Med J 2009;68(2):27–9.

34. Couppié P, Domergue V, Clyti E, et al. Increased incidence of leprosy following HAART initiation: a manifestation of the immune reconstitution disease. AIDS 2009;23(12):1599–600.

35. Desjeux P, Alvar J. Leishmania/HIV co-infections: epidemiology in Europe. Ann Trop Med Parasitol 2003;97:S3–15.

36. Posada-Vergara MP, Lindoso JA, Tolezano JE, et al. Tegumentary leishmaniasis as a manifestation of immune reconstitution inflammatory syndrome in 2 patients with AIDS. J Infect Dis 2005;192:1819–22.

37. Chrusciak-Talhari A, Ribeiro-Rodrigues R, Talhari C, et al. Case report: tegumentary leishmaniasis as the cause of immune reconstitution inflammatory syndrome in a patient co-infected with human immunodeficiency virus and Leishmania guyanensis. Am J Trop Med Hyg 2009;81(4):559–64.

38. Sinha S, Fernandez G, Kapila R, et al. Diffuse cutaneous leishmaniasis associated with the immune reconstitution inflammatory syndrome. Int J Dermatol 2008;47:1263–70.

39. Gelanew T, Amogne W, Abebe T, et al. A clinical isolate of Leishmania donovani with ITS1 sequence polymorphism as a cause of para-kala-azar dermal leishmaniasis in an Ethiopian human immunodeficiency virus–positive patient on highly active antiretroviral therapy. Br J Dermatol 2010;163(4):870–4.

40. Ridolfo AL, Gervasoni C, Antinori S, et al. Post-kala-azar dermal leishmaniasis during highly active antiretroviral therapy in an AIDS patient infected with Leishmania infantum. J Infect 2000;40(2):199–202.

41. Gilad J, Borer A, Hallel-Halevy D, et al. Post-kala-azar dermal leishmaniasis manifesting after initiation of highly active anti-retroviral therapy in a patient with human immunodeficiency virus infection. Isr Med Assoc J 2001;3(6):451–2.

42. Tadesse A, Hurissa Z. Leishmaniasis (PKDL) as a case of immune reconstitution inflammatory syndrome (IRIS) in HIV-positive patient after initiation of anti-retroviral therapy (ART). Ethiop Med J 2009; 47(1):77–9.

43. Belay AD, Asafa Y, Mesure J, et al. Successful miltefosine treatment of post-kala-azar dermal leishmaniasis occurring during antiretroviral therapy. Ann Trop Med Parasitol 2006;100(3):223–7.

44. Antinori S, Longhi E, Bestetti G, et al. Post-kala-azar dermal leishmaniasis as an immune reconstitution inflammatory syndrome in a patient with acquired immune deficiency syndrome. Br J Dermatol 2007; 157(5):1032–6.

45. Kerob D, Bouaziz JD, Sarfati C, et al. First case of cutaneous reconstitution inflammatory syndrome with HIV infection and leishmaniasis. Clin Infect Dis 2006;43:664–6.

46. Gupta S, Mathur P, Maskey D, et al. Immune restoration syndrome with disseminated Penicillium marneffei and cytomegalovirus co-infections in an AIDS patient. AIDS Res Ther 2007;4:21.

47. Saikia L, Nath R, Hazarika D, et al. Atypical cutaneous lesions of Penicillium marneffei infection as a manifestation of the immune reconstitution inflammatory syndrome after highly active antiretroviral therapy. Indian J Dermatol Venereol Leprol 2010; 76:45–8.

48. Saikia L, Nath R, Biswanath P, et al. infection in HIV infected patients in Nagaland and immune reconstitution after treatment. Indian J Med Res 2009;129:333–4.

49. Gutierrez-Galhardo MC, Francesconi do Valle AC, Barros Fraga BL, et al. Disseminated sporotrichosis as a manifestation of immune reconstitution inflammatory syndrome. Mycoses 2008;53:78–80.

50. Lanzafame M, Faggian F, Lattuada E, et al. Strongyloidiasis in an HIV-1-infected patient after highly active antiretroviral therapy-induced immune restoration. J Infect Dis 2005;191:1026–7.

Arsenical Keratoses in Bangladesh—Update and Prevention Strategies

Arlene M. Ruiz de Luzuriaga, MD, MPH[a],*,
Habibul Ahsan, MD, MMedSc[b], Christopher R. Shea, MD[a]

KEYWORDS

• Arsenicosis • Bangladesh • Skin cancer • Keratoses

Arsenic contamination of drinking water in Bangladesh has been called the "largest mass poisoning of a population in history,"[1] a consequence of the widespread installation and use of tube wells intended to provide a safer alternative to surface water sources that could easily be contaminated by microorganisms. It has been estimated that by the 1990s, 95% of the rural population of Bangladesh was drinking water from tube wells.[2]

The current World Health Organization (WHO) guideline designates 0.01 mg/L as the maximum permissible amount of arsenic in drinking water. The National Arsenic Mitigation Information Center reported in 2008 that of 4.8 million tube wells evaluated by field testing kits in Bangladesh, almost 30% had arsenic levels exceeding 0.05 mg/L.[3] This inorganic arsenic contamination is of natural origin, with arsenic thought to be released to the groundwater from the surrounding sediment.[4,5] A recent survey by Chakraborti and colleagues[6] estimated that in Bangladesh, 36 million people are at risk of drinking arsenic-contaminated water at arsenic levels more than 0.01 mg/L, with 22 million at risk of drinking water with arsenic levels more than 0.05 mg/L. Previous estimates put the population at risk for arsenic exposure at levels beyond the WHO guideline to be as much as 35 million to 57 million.[7,8]

Chronic arsenicosis is defined by the WHO as a "chronic health condition arising from prolonged ingestion of arsenic above a safe dose for at least 6 months, usually manifested by characteristic skin lesions of melanosis and keratosis, occurring alone or in combination, with or without involvement of internal organs."[9] The latency for the appearance of clinical signs and symptoms of chronic exposure can range from 6 to 10 months or even 20 years or more.[10,11] Extracutaneous manifestations include neurologic changes, hypertension and cardiovascular disease, pulmonary disease, peripheral vascular disease, diabetes, adverse pregnancy outcomes, and internal malignancy.[12,13] Arsenic is considered a Class I human carcinogen by the International Agency for Research on Cancer because of its increased risk for skin cancer, as well as internal cancers, such as lung and bladder cancer.[14] Proposed mechanisms for arsenic carcinogenesis include chromosome abnormalities, oxidative stress, altered growth factors, cell proliferation, promotion and/or progression in carcinogenesis, altered DNA repair, p53 gene suppression, altered DNA methylation patterns, and gene amplification.[15,16]

The authors have nothing to disclose.
[a] Section of Dermatology, Department of Medicine, University of Chicago Medical Center, 5841 South Maryland Avenue, Mail Code 5067, L502, Chicago, IL 60637, USA
[b] Departments of Medicine and Human Genetics and Cancer Research Center, University of Chicago, 5841 South Maryland Avenue N102, Chicago, IL 60637, USA
* Corresponding author.
E-mail address: arlene.ruizdeluzuriaga@uchospitals.edu

Dermatol Clin 29 (2011) 45–51
doi:10.1016/j.det.2010.09.003

derm.theclinics.com

At very high concentrations of exposure, systemic symptoms, most commonly gastrointestinal symptoms as well as peripheral neuropathy, may precede skin lesions.[17] Recently evaluated data from the Health Effects of Arsenic Longitudinal Study (HEALS) show that the risk of all-cause mortality and chronic disease mortality increased with increasing arsenic exposure, particularly long-term exposure.[18]

CUTANEOUS DISEASE

The first case of arsenicosis was identified in a patient in Bangladesh as early as 1984,[19] and a recent study found patients with skin lesions in 31 of 33 surveyed districts in Bangladesh.[6] Arsenic-related skin lesions are considered the earliest manifestation of nonmalignant disease related to chronic arsenic exposure.[20] The risk for nonmalignant and malignant skin disease seems to increase with increasing dose.[20,21] One study noted that subjects exposed to an arsenic concentration of 0.05 mg/L had a 59% higher risk of skin lesions compared with unexposed subjects.[22] Skin changes can be found with chronic exposure to nonlethal doses of arsenic, ranging from 0.005 to 0.09 mg/kg/d.[9]

Nonmalignant and Premalignant Disease

Of the skin findings occurring in arsenicosis, pigmentary changes are considered to be the earliest dermatologic findings. These alterations can be diffuse or patchy and are often localized to the palms and soles. Characteristic patterns include a freckled raindrop pattern, leucomelanosis (guttate hypopigmentation in a background of hyperpigmentation), and mucosal pigmentation. Conjunctival congestion and nonpitting edema have also been demonstrated.[10]

The presence of arsenical keratoses has been suggested to be a sensitive marker for early detection of arsenicosis and is the most common manifestation preceding the development of arsenic-related skin cancer.[23,24] Typical lesions are hyperkeratotic, punctate, firm papules measuring 2 to 10 mm in diameter and are often located at sites subject to friction or trauma (**Fig. 1**). Common locations are the palms and soles, although they may also be present on the dorsal surface of the extremities[25,26]; other locations include the trunk, genitalia, and eyelids. Arsenical keratoses also may present as scaly, erythematous, or hyperpigmented plaques. Thickened leathery plaques may have associated hyperhidrosis. The extent of disease is graded on a scale of mild, moderate, and severe. In mild disease, lesions are usually less than 2 mm in

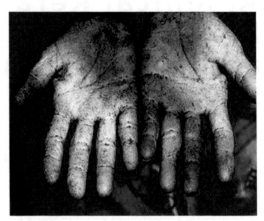

Fig. 1. Arsenical keratoses involving the palms.

diameter and are most easily found by palpation. Involved skin may be indurated, with a gritlike character. Moderate disease is characterized by raised lesions ranging from 2 to 5 mm in diameter, with punctate or wartlike features. Findings in severe disease include lesions more than 5 mm in diameter, which may coalesce into plaques with subsequent cracking and fissuring of the skin.[9,26] In contrast to arsenic-related internal malignancies with long latent periods to manifestation, premalignant arsenical keratoses may appear after only a brief time of arsenic exposure.[10] An erythematous halo around the keratoses or a thickening may indicate progression to in situ squamous cell carcinoma (SCC).[27] In addition, bleeding and a sudden increase in cracking, fissuring, or size are suggestive of malignant transformation.[28] The presence of arsenical keratosis may also mandate further screening for internal malignancy.[29] Patients with large, thickened lesions may experience discomfort, particularly because of secondary fissuring and cracking, and they are at increased risk for subsequent infection.[3] Social stigmatization can occur as the cutaneous manifestations of arsenicosis are sometimes incorrectly thought to indicate a contagious disease, leading to marital discord, employment difficulties, and social isolation.[28,30,31] Other cutaneous diseases that should be included in the differential diagnosis for the skin findings in arsenicosis are listed in **Table 1**.

Malignant Disease

Cutaneous malignancies resulting from arsenic exposure include in situ and invasive SCC (**Fig. 2**), basal cell carcinoma (BCC), and less often, Merkel cell carcinoma.[32–35] These malignancies usually develop 10 to 20 years after the initial manifestation of arsenicosis, often as large

Table 1
Differential diagnosis of cutaneous findings in arsenicosis

Primary Skin Finding	Differential Diagnosis
Diffuse melanosis	Ashy dermatosis, actinic dermatosis, melasma, drug-induced hyperpigmentation, acanthosis nigricans, chronic liver disorders, porphyria cutanea tarda, Wilson disease
Guttate (spotted) melanosis	Pityriasis versicolor, solar or simple lentigines, lichen planus, drug-induced hyperpigmentation, xeroderma pigmentosum, Peutz-Jeghers syndrome, post-kala-azar dermal leishmaniasis
Leucomelanosis	Idiopathic guttate hypomelanosis, pityriasis versicolor, pityriasis lichenoides chronica, leprosy, post-kala-azar dermal leishmaniasis
Diffuse keratosis	Palmoplantar psoriasis, atopic dermatitis, frictional/occupational keratosis, tinea pedum, pitted keratolysis, genetic keratodermas and ichthyoses, discoid lupus erythematosus, pityriasis rubra pilaris
Nodular/Spotted keratosis	Frictional/occupational keratosis, verruca vulgaris, corn/callus, seborrheic keratosis, epidermodysplasia verruciformis

Data from Caussy D, editor. A field guide for detection, management, and surveillance of arsenicosis cases. New Delhi (India): World Health Organization, Regional Office of South-East Asia; 2005. p. 1–38; and Saha KC. Diagnosis of arsenicosis. J Environ Sci Health A Tox Hazard Subst Environ Eng 2003;38:255–72.

keratotic nodules.[19] In contrast to the typical sun-exposed distribution of most nonmelanomatous skin cancers, those resulting from arsenic exposure tend to occur in nonexposed sites.[33] In addition, the malignancies may be multiple and can arise both in areas of existing keratoses and in uninvolved skin. Invasive SCC that develops within keratoses in patients with a history of

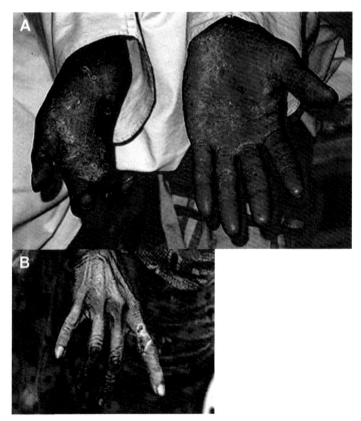

Fig. 2. (*A, B*) SCC affecting the hands.

arsenic exposure may be aggressive with a heightened metastatic risk.[17] BCCs arising in the setting of arsenic exposure tend to be multiple and may resemble in situ SCC clinically.[17]

Risk Factors

Several studies have indicated that men are more susceptible to the arsenic-related skin effects than women, a finding that may be explained by metabolism.[23,36–38] A population-based study in Bangladesh showed a strong association between more efficient methylation of arsenic and decreased risk of developing skin lesions in women as compared with men.[38] Additional risk factors for skin lesions include tobacco use, sun exposure, increasing age, folate deficiency, hyperhomocysteinemia, and low urinary creatinine excretion.[32,36,39–43] Genetic variability affecting the metabolic capacity of arsenic also contributes to risk for skin lesions.[44–46]

Laboratory Findings

Arsenic exposure can be established by testing environmental sources, such as the water being consumed, and by monitoring the patient. Biologic monitoring as a measure of arsenic exposure most commonly includes measuring arsenic concentration in urine, hair, nail, and serum. Urine is the primary route of elimination of most arsenic species. Spot urine samples are taken commonly, being easy and painless to collect.[47] Previous data have suggested that the level of arsenic in urine does not vary significantly over time and can be used as a long-term biomarker of arsenic exposure provided that the exposure is current and ongoing.[21,24] Urine samples taken more than 24 to 48 hours after the last exposure can underestimate peak exposure because most of the arsenic would have been excreted. In addition, the subject should not have consumed any seafood for 4 days before urine collection.[48] Hair and nail samples can be useful to estimate the average amount and rate of arsenic exposure within the previous 9 months.[49] However, these samples can be influenced by external contamination by environmental arsenic exposure.[50] According to the WHO 2005 field guide for the detection of arsenicosis, a urine sample with arsenic concentration greater than 50 μg/L confirms recent exposure. Dry hair with a concentration greater than 1 mg/kg or nail with a concentration greater than 1.5 mg/kg may indicate of exposure to unsafe doses of arsenic within the previous 11 months.[9] Serum concentrations are not so commonly used to screen for chronic exposure because arsenic is rapidly cleared from the blood; serum testing is most useful to assess recent high-concentration exposures.[48]

Histologically, premalignant and malignant, cutaneous, arsenic-related tumors are generally indistinguishable from their counterparts due to ultraviolet radiation. Together with clinical and social history, the absence of significant dermal solar elastosis may be a helpful clue to identify the cause. Arsenical keratoses typically demonstrate compact parakeratosis overlying an acanthotic epidermis with mild keratinocytic dysplasia. There may also be some basal keratinocyte vacuolization and a chronic inflammatory dermal infiltrate.[10,51] As in non-arsenic–related SCC in situ, full-thickness intraepidermal atypia with parakeratotic hyperkeratosis, without invasion of the dermis, characterizes arsenic-related SCC in situ. When BCC is caused by arsenic, it is usually of the superficial pattern; however, nodular, reticulated, and pigmented patterns of BCC may all be associated with chronic arsenic exposure.[27,52] Arsenic-related BCCs may demonstrate vacuolated cells, dyskeratosis, multinucleated giant cells, and increased numbers of atypical nuclei and mitotic figures.[17,52]

Management and Prevention

Management and prevention of the cutaneous sequelae of chronic arsenic exposure is multifaceted. Symptomatic treatment of arsenical keratoses with or without pigmentary changes includes the use of topical 5% to 10% salicylic acid and 10% to 20% urea ointment.[9] Treatment of arsenic-related cutaneous neoplasms includes surgical excision, cryosurgery, electrodesiccation and curettage, oral retinoid therapy, and topical chemotherapy.[53–56] Imiquimod 5% cream used once daily for 6 weeks has been found effective against arsenical keratoses, SCCs, and BCCs.[54,55] Dietary modifications and vitamin supplementation to influence the methylation and subsequent detoxification of arsenic have been found to reduce the deleterious effects of arsenic on the skin. These measures include supplementation with vitamin E, selenium,[57] folic acid,[41] riboflavin, and pyridoxine, with the effects of the B vitamins possibly being additive.[22] The levels at which such nutrients need to be consumed to have a beneficial effect are greater than the current recommended daily amounts.[22] Studies have also confirmed that a lower body mass index is associated with a higher prevalence of skin lesions, supporting that overall malnutrition may increase the risk for arsenic-related skin disease.[39,58] Chelation therapy with agents such as dimercaptosuccinic acid, dimercaptopropane succinate, and D-penicillamine has variable benefits for patients with chronic arsenicosis.[28]

Cessation of consuming contaminated water is of utmost importance. Arsenic mitigation efforts are underway to address this pressing issue. Interventions that have been implemented include person-to-person reporting of well test results, well labeling, village and individual health education, and installation of more deeply situated wells; in Bangladesh, at least 350-m deep aquifers have been found to be safe from arsenic contamination.[6] In one study, urinary arsenic levels decreased by 46% in people who switched to a well identified as safe.[59] Other proposals to decrease consumption of arsenic-contaminated water include rainwater harvesting, filtration and removal of arsenic from current water supplies via individual devices or treatment plants, and treatment of surface water with pressure filtration and disinfection.[9]

Arsenical keratoses and their sequelae are significant contributors to morbidity resulting from chronic exposure to arsenic in drinking water in Bangladesh and they may also serve as indicators for further systemic evaluation for disease. It is to be hoped that a combination of mitigation proposals and programs with surveillance by the medical community for latent sequelae and public health education and counseling will mitigate the deadly impact of chronic arsenic exposure in this population and guide future efforts worldwide.

REFERENCES

1. Smith AH, Lingas EO, Rahman M. Contamination of drinking-water by arsenic in Bangladesh: a public health emergency. Bull World Health Organ 2000; 78(9):1093–103.

2. Caldwell BK, Caldwell JC, Mitra SN, et al. Searching for an optimum solution to the Bangladesh arsenic crisis. Soc Sci Med 2003;56(10):2089–96.

3. UNICEF. Arsenic mitigation in Bangladesh. Available at: http://www.unicef.org/bangladesh/Arsenic.pdf. Accessed July 31, 2010.

4. British Geological Survey. Arsenic contamination of groundwater: Bangladesh phase 1. Available at: http://www.bgs.ac.uk/arsenic/bphase1/b_intro.htm. Accessed July 31, 2010.

5. Ng JC, Wang J, Shraim A. A global health problem caused by arsenic from natural sources. Chemosphere 2003;52(9):1353–9.

6. Chakraborti D, Rahman MM, Das B, et al. Status of groundwater arsenic contamination in Bangladesh: a 14-year study report. Water Res 2010. [Epub ahead of print].

7. Ahsan H, Perrin M, Rahman A, et al. Associations between drinking water and urinary arsenic levels and skin lesions in Bangladesh. J Occup Environ Med 2000;42(12):1195–201.

8. Smith MM, Hore T, Chakraborty P, et al. A dugwell program to provide arsenic-safe water in West Bengal, India: preliminary results. J Environ Sci Health A Tox Hazard Subst Environ Eng 2003;38(1):289–99.

9. Caussy D, editor. A field guide for detection, management, and surveillance of arsenicosis cases. New Delhi (India): World Health Organization, Regional Office of South-East Asia; 2005. p. 1–38.

10. Saha KC. Diagnosis of arsenicosis. J Environ Sci Health A Tox Hazard Subst Environ Eng 2003; 38(1):255–72.

11. Haque R, Mazumder DN, Samanta S, et al. Arsenic in drinking water and skin lesions: dose-response data from West Bengal, India. Epidemiology 2003; 14(2):174–82.

12. Waalkes MP, Liu J, Germolec DR, et al. Arsenic exposure in utero exacerbates skin cancer response in adulthood with contemporaneous distortion of tumor stem cell dynamics. Cancer Res 2008; 68(20):8278–85.

13. von Ehrenstein OS, Guha Mazumder DN, Hira-Smith M, et al. Pregnancy outcomes, infant mortality, and arsenic in drinking water in West Bengal, India. Am J Epidemiol 2006;163(7):662–9.

14. An evaluation of chemicals and industrial processes associated with cancer in humans based on human and animal data: IARC Monographs Volumes 1 to 20. Report of an IARC Working Group. Cancer Res 1980;40(1):1–12.

15. Kitchin KT. Recent advances in arsenic carcinogenesis: modes of action, animal model systems, and methylated arsenic metabolites. Toxicol Appl Pharmacol 2001;172(3):249–61.

16. Germolec DR, Spalding J, Yu HS, et al. Arsenic enhancement of skin neoplasia by chronic stimulation of growth factors. Am J Pathol 1998;153(6): 1775–85.

17. Schwartz RA. Arsenic and the skin. Int J Dermatol 1997;36(4):241–50.

18. Argos M, Kalra T, Rathouz PJ, et al. Arsenic exposure from drinking water, and all-cause and chronic-disease mortalities in Bangladesh (HEALS): a prospective cohort study. Lancet 2010;376(9737): 252–8.

19. Saha KC. Cutaneous malignancy in arsenicosis. Br J Dermatol 2001;145(1):185.

20. Yoshida T, Yamauchi H, Fan Sun G. Chronic health effects in people exposed to arsenic via the drinking water: dose-response relationships in review. Toxicol Appl Pharmacol 2004;198(3):243–52.

21. Chen Y, Parvez F, Gamble M, et al. Arsenic exposure at low-to-moderate levels and skin lesions, arsenic metabolism, neurological functions, and biomarkers for respiratory and cardiovascular diseases: review of recent findings from the Health Effects of Arsenic

Longitudinal Study (HEALS) in Bangladesh. Toxicol Appl Pharmacol 2009;239(2):184–92.

22. Zablotska LB, Chen Y, Graziano JH, et al. Protective effects of B vitamins and antioxidants on the risk of arsenic-related skin lesions in Bangladesh. Environ Health Perspect 2008;116(8):1056–62.

23. Kadono T, Inaoka T, Murayama N, et al. Skin manifestations of arsenicosis in two villages in Bangladesh. Int J Dermatol 2002;41(12):841–6.

24. Tseng WP, Chu HM, How SW, et al. Prevalence of skin cancer in an endemic area of chronic arsenicism in Taiwan. J Natl Cancer Inst 1968;40(3): 453–63.

25. Sengupta MK, Mukherjee A, Hossain MA, et al. Groundwater arsenic contamination in the Ganga-Padma-Meghna-Brahmaputra plain of India and Bangladesh. Arch Environ Health 2003;58(11): 701–2.

26. Sengupta SR, Das NK, Datta PK. Pathogenesis, clinical features and pathology of chronic arsenicosis. Indian J Dermatol Venereol Leprol 2008;74(6): 559–70.

27. Schwartz RA. Premalignant keratinocytic neoplasms. J Am Acad Dermatol 1996;35(2 Pt 1): 223–42.

28. Das NK, Sengupta SR. Arsenicosis: diagnosis and treatment. Indian J Dermatol Venereol Leprol 2008; 74(6):571–81.

29. Cuzick J, Sasieni P, Evans S. Ingested arsenic, keratoses, and bladder cancer. Am J Epidemiol 1992; 136(4):417–21.

30. Ahmad SA, Sayed MH, Khan MH, et al. Sociocultural aspects of arsenicosis in Bangladesh: community perspective. J Environ Sci Health A Tox Hazard Subst Environ Eng 2007;42(12):1945–58.

31. Hassan MM, Atkins PJ, Dunn CE. Social implications of arsenic poisoning in Bangladesh. Soc Sci Med 2005;61(10):2201–11.

32. Elmariah SB, Anolik R, Walters RF, et al. Invasive squamous-cell carcinoma and arsenical keratoses. Dermatol Online J 2008;14(10):24.

33. Boonchai W, Green A, Ng J, et al. Basal cell carcinoma in chronic arsenicism occurring in Queensland, Australia, after ingestion of an asthma medication. J Am Acad Dermatol 2000;43(4):664–9.

34. Wong SS, Tan KC, Goh CL. Cutaneous manifestations of chronic arsenicism: review of seventeen cases. J Am Acad Dermatol 1998;38(2 Pt 1): 179–85.

35. Lien HC, Tsai TF, Lee YY, et al. Merkel cell carcinoma and chronic arsenicism. J Am Acad Dermatol 1999; 41(4):641–3.

36. Rahman M, Vahter M, Sohel N, et al. Arsenic exposure and age and sex-specific risk for skin lesions: a population-based case-referent study in Bangladesh. Environ Health Perspect 2006; 114(12):1847–52.

37. Vahter M, Concha G. Role of metabolism in arsenic toxicity. Pharmacol Toxicol 2001;89(1):1–5.

38. Lindberg AL, Rahman M, Persson LA, et al. The risk of arsenic induced skin lesions in Bangladeshi men and women is affected by arsenic metabolism and the age at first exposure. Toxicol Appl Pharmacol 2008;230(1):9–16.

39. Ahsan H, Chen Y, Parvez F, et al. Arsenic exposure from drinking water and risk of premalignant skin lesions in Bangladesh: baseline results from the Health Effects of Arsenic Longitudinal Study. Am J Epidemiol 2006;163(12):1138–48.

40. Chen Y, Graziano JH, Parvez F, et al. Modification of risk of arsenic-induced skin lesions by sunlight exposure, smoking, and occupational exposures in Bangladesh. Epidemiology 2006;17(4):459–67.

41. Gamble MV, Liu X, Ahsan H, et al. Folate, homocysteine, and arsenic metabolism in arsenic-exposed individuals in Bangladesh. Environ Health Perspect 2005;113(12):1683–8.

42. Lindberg AL, Sohel N, Rahman M, et al. Impact of smoking and chewing tobacco on arsenic-induced skin lesions. Environ Health Perspect 2010;118(4): 533–8.

43. Pilsner JR, Liu X, Ahsan H, et al. Folate deficiency, hyperhomocysteinemia, low urinary creatinine, and hypomethylation of leukocyte DNA are risk factors for arsenic-induced skin lesions. Environ Health Perspect 2009;117(2):254–60.

44. Argos M, Kibriya MG, Parvez F, et al. Gene expression profiles in peripheral lymphocytes by arsenic exposure and skin lesion status in a Bangladeshi population. Cancer Epidemiol Biomarkers Prev 2006;15(7):1367–75.

45. De Chaudhuri S, Ghosh P, Sarma N, et al. Genetic variants associated with arsenic susceptibility: study of purine nucleoside phosphorylase, arsenic (+3) methyltransferase, and glutathione S-transferase omega genes. Environ Health Perspect 2008; 116(4):501–5.

46. Hernandez A, Marcos R. Genetic variations associated with interindividual sensitivity in the response to arsenic exposure. Pharmacogenomics 2008; 9(8):1113–32.

47. Calderon RL, Hudgens E, Le XC, et al. Excretion of arsenic in urine as a function of exposure to arsenic in drinking water. Environ Health Perspect 1999; 107(8):663–7.

48. Orloff K, Mistry K, Metcalf S. Biomonitoring for environmental exposures to arsenic. J Toxicol Environ Health B Crit Rev 2009;12(7):509–24.

49. Kile ML, Houseman EA, Breton CV, et al. Association between total ingested arsenic and toenail arsenic concentrations. J Environ Sci Health A Tox Hazard Subst Environ Eng 2007;42(12):1827–34.

50. Karagas MR. Arsenic-related mortality in Bangladesh. Lancet 2010;376(9737):213–4.

51. Yeh S. Skin cancer in chronic arsenicism. Hum Pathol 1973;4(4):469—85.

52. Yeh S, How SW, Lin CS. Arsenical cancer of skin. Histologic study with special reference to Bowen's disease. Cancer 1968;21(2):312—39.

53. Watson K, Creamer D. Arsenic-induced keratoses and Bowen's disease. Clin Exp Dermatol 2004; 29(1):46—8.

54. Lonergan CL, McNamara EK, Cordoro KM, et al. Imiquimod cream 5% for the treatment of arsenic-induced cutaneous neoplasms. Cutis 2010; 85(4):199—202.

55. Boonchai W. Treatment of precancerous and cancerous lesions of chronic arsenicism with 5% imiquimod cream. Arch Dermatol 2006;142(4): 531—2.

56. Yerebakan O, Ermis O, Yilmaz E, et al. Treatment of arsenical keratosis and Bowen's disease with acitretin. Int J Dermatol 2002;41(2):84—7.

57. Verret WJ, Chen Y, Ahmed A, et al. A randomized, double-blind placebo-controlled trial evaluating the effects of vitamin E and selenium on arsenic-induced skin lesions in Bangladesh. J Occup Environ Med 2005;47(10):1026—35.

58. Guha Mazumder DN, Haque R, Ghosh N, et al. Arsenic levels in drinking water and the prevalence of skin lesions in West Bengal, India. Int J Epidemiol 1998;27(5):871—7.

59. Chen Y, van Geen A, Graziano JH, et al. Reduction in urinary arsenic levels in response to arsenic mitigation efforts in Araihazar, Bangladesh. Environ Health Perspect 2007;115(6):917—23.

Chagas Disease: Coming to a Place Near You

Eva Rawlings Parker, MD[a],*, Aisha Sethi, MD[b]

KEYWORDS

- Chagas disease • *Trypanosoma cruzi*
- American trypanosomiasis

Chagas disease, or American trypanosomiasis, is a parasitic infection caused by the flagellate protozoan *Trypanosoma cruzi*, an organism that is endemic to Latin America. This disease was first described in 1909 by the Brazilian physician Carlos Chagas, and today the World Health Organization (WHO) estimates that approximately 10 million people are infected.[1]

Although not formally identified until 100 years ago, more recent paleoparasitology studies have revealed the presence of *T cruzi* DNA in tissue from 9000-year-old pre-Colombian mummies, providing a historical glimpse into an illness that has likely plagued humans for thousands of years and continues to have significant morbidity and mortality and impose far-reaching socioeconomic effects.[2]

TRANSMISSION

Chagas disease is primarily a vector-borne illness, with most infections transmitted by blood-sucking reduviid bugs, members of the insect subfamily Triatominae.[3] Triatomines live in the cracks and crevices of poorly constructed mud and thatch homes and emerge at night to procure their blood meal. Most bites are therefore incurred while sleeping and commonly occur on the exposed skin of the face, hence the insects' common name, kissing bugs. The parasite is transmitted when infected fecal matter from the insect is inoculated into mucosal surfaces or minor breaks in the skin.[4] Within this subfamily, *Triatoma infestans*, *Rhodnius prolixus*, and *Triatoma dimidiata* serve

as the 3 most important vectors of human infection. Chagas disease has remained a prolific infectious disease partly because of its large number of mammalian reservoirs, with more than 150 species of domestic, farm, and wild animals (cats, dogs, pigs, rodents, marsupials, armadillos) confirmed as carriers of *T cruzi*.[3]

Alternate modes of transmission include blood transfusions, solid organ and bone marrow transplants, congenital infection from vertical maternal-fetal transmission, oral infection through food-borne contamination, and rarely, by accidental laboratory exposure.[3,5–13]

Historically, transfusion of contaminated blood products has been a common and well-recognized source of *T cruzi* infections in Latin America.[14] In contrast, only 7 cases of transfusion-associated Chagas disease, all in immunocompromised patients, have been documented in the last 2 decades for the United States and Canada combined.[5,7] However, the Centers for Disease Control and Prevention (CDC) have reported that nearly 800 cases of Chagas disease have been confirmed in donors at blood donation centers in the United States since 2007, when voluntary screening for this infection was first introduced. Although most of these cases have been concentrated where large populations of Latin American immigrants live, such as California, Texas, Florida, and New York, donor positivity has been documented in 42 states within the contiguous United States.[7,15]

Similarly, the number of confirmed transplant-associated cases of Chagas disease in the United

The authors have nothing to disclose.
a Franklin Dermatology Group, 740 Cool Springs Boulevard, Suite 200, Franklin, TN 37067, USA
b Section of Dermatology, University of Chicago Medical Center, 5841 South Maryland Avenue, MC 5067, Chicago, IL 60637, USA
* Corresponding author.
E-mail address: evaparker@yahoo.com

Dermatol Clin 29 (2011) 53–62
doi:10.1016/j.det.2010.08.011

derm.theclinics.com

States also remains small. However, reports of both new infections and reactivation of previous disease have been documented in patients receiving cardiac, renal, and other solid organ and bone marrow transplants in Latin America and represent a growing concern in nonendemic areas.[8–10,16–21]

Another important source of *T cruzi* infection in both endemic and nonendemic regions is transplacental transmission, with 1 in 20 neonates born to seropositive mothers being diagnosed with congenital Chagas disease.[12,22] In addition to the concern for congenital infection, Chagas disease also increases the risk of spontaneous abortion and prematurity. Whereas prevention of vertical transmission is not possible, early detection of infection in neonates and prompt treatment greatly reduces the morbidity and mortality.[12]

Although suspected for decades as a potential source of infection, outbreaks of food-borne Chagas disease have been confirmed in recent years in Latin America and are largely linked to contamination of food with fecal matter from triatomine insects. Typically, raw meat or juices derived from sugarcane, guava, or acai berries have been implicated in the oral transmission of *T cruzi*.[23–25]

Whereas these modes of transmission represent the minority of cases of Chagas disease, nonvectorial routes are emerging as important sources of new infections, especially in nonendemic regions worldwide.

Epidemiology and Economic Effect

Historically, Chagas disease has affected impoverished rural populations in Mexico and Central and South America, where shoddy construction of domiciles allows the triatomine vectors to thrive.[26] Increasingly, however, Chagas disease is being identified in major cities throughout Latin America, largely a consequence of urbanization and the migration of rural people into metropolitan areas.[27]

The WHO classifies Chagas disease as a neglected tropical disease. This designation implies that the transmission of infection is propagated by poverty, and that the disease often affects vulnerable populations, including indigenous and rural groups, women, children, and the elderly. Furthermore, because poverty favors a greater burden of disease, the large economic effect of this disease in turn contributes to further promoting poverty.[28–30] Indeed, the economic burden of this disease is significant. In many Latin American countries, the direct and indirect costs, including the cost of health care in dollars and loss of productivity, attributable to Chagas disease ranges from $40 million to in excess of $800 million per nation per annum. Furthermore, as a whole, Latin America experiences economic losses totaling $18 billion annually as a result of the early morbidity and mortality associated with Chagas disease.[31]

An estimated 18 million natives of Mexico and Central and South America have migrated into the United States.[15] Because of this large influx of Latin American immigrants, the CDC estimates that at least 300,000 people currently living within United States are infected with Chagas disease.[32] While most cases of Chagas disease reported in the United States are imported from the endemic regions by immigrants or travelers or transmitted by nonvectorial routes, a handful of vector-transmitted autochthonous infections have been documented in the United States.[33,34] In fact, triatomine insects are abundant in the Southern United States. A recent study demonstrated that 41% of the insects collected from in and around the homes in Tucson, Arizona were infected with *T cruzi*, illustrating that the risk of vector-borne transmission of Chagas disease within the United States may be greater than that previously perceived.[34] In addition, several animal reservoirs also exist in many Southern states, evidenced by the identification of *T cruzi* infection in 20 species of wildlife, particularly raccoons and possums.[35,36] Of greater concern is the growing number of documented cases of Chagas disease in canines, with numerous cases now reported in dogs from Texas, Tennessee, Louisiana, Oklahoma, Georgia, South Carolina, and Virginia, demonstrating that an active canine transmission cycle for *T cruzi* exists in the United States. Many features of canine infection parallel the clinical findings in humans, and consequently, Chagas disease confers significant morbidity and mortality on dogs that become infected, requiring veterinarians to increase their recognition of this disease.[37–42]

Because of the effect of globalization on immigration patterns coupled with the poor recognition of this infection in nonendemic regions and a lack of mandatory screening for all blood and tissue donors, Chagas disease will likely become a growing health threat in the United States. As a result, the current epidemiology of this disease is likely to evolve considerably over the coming decades.[14,16,43,44]

PATHOGENESIS

The prolific and persistent nature of Chagas disease is likely multifactorial. Without question, the socioeconomic factors, including poverty and substandard housing in rural Latin America, have played a significant role. However, other unique aspects of this parasite's biology have also contributed, including its large number of mammalian reservoirs, the parasite's genetic heterogeneity, and a complex cascade of T cruzi-host cell interactions.[3,45]

Although considerable research effort has focused on these interactions, large gaps in the understanding of T cruzi pathogenesis remain and conflicting theories persist.[46,47] Most agree that parasite persistence plays an integral role in this disease. Obviously, many complex interactions between the host and parasite dictate the immunopathology of Chagas disease and determine the outcome and success of T cruzi persistence in the human host.[3,47,48] For example, molecular mimicry, which promotes autoimmunity,[49] overexpression of parasite peroxiredoxins to counter the host's oxidative assault,[50] and overexpression of parasitic cysteine proteases such as cruzipain, which trigger a cascade of molecular events resulting in inflammation and tissue damage,[47,51] are mechanisms that favor parasite persistence. Conversely, a robust T helper cell 1 immune response by the host results in the production of key cytokines, including interferon γ, tumor necrosis factor α, and interleukin 12, along with nitric oxide, which is trypanocidal, and serves to effectively reduce parasite load.[3,52,53] Ultimately, the complex web of specific pathways involved in the parasite pathogenesis and human immunopathology of Chagas disease is yet to be fully elucidated, and therefore much of the molecular mystery regarding this infection persists.[47]

Clinical Presentation

Infection with T cruzi has 2 phases: acute and chronic. The acute phase lasts 4 to 8 weeks and is asymptomatic in most infected individuals but may also present as a self-limited febrile illness. If symptomatic, acute Chagas disease manifests as a flulike illness within 1 to 2 weeks of exposure and typically presents with prolonged fever, malaise, anorexia, nausea, vomiting, and diarrhea. When more serious, the patient may display hepatosplenomegaly, lymphadenopathy, and edema. In addition, abnormalities on electrocardiogram (ECG) or cardiomegaly on chest radiograph may be observed, and in rare instances myocarditis, meningoencephalitis, or pneumonitis may develop. Deaths due to acute Chagas disease are seen in less than 10% of symptomatic cases and are attributable to these more severe complications. The risk for fulminant presentations is increased in newborns with congenital infection, children, and immunocompromised individuals.[3]

Of particular note are the local inflammatory reactions at the sites of inoculation, which serve as the earliest and most specific mucocutaneous manifestations of Chagas disease. At cutaneous sites of inoculation, a violaceous, indurated, furuncular nodule with discrete central edema known as a chagoma may develop. If inoculation occurs via the conjunctival mucosae, the patient rapidly develops asymptomatic, unilateral, bipalpebral edema and conjunctivitis with ipsilateral regional lymphadenopathy, a constellation of findings referred to as Romaña sign or ophthalmoganglionar complex. This condition may be complicated by the subsequent development of periorbital cellulitis and metastatic chagomas. Chagomas may persist for several weeks before spontaneously resolving. Finally, a nonspecific and transient morbilliform or urticarial exanthem called schizotripanides may also be observed in the acute phase of the illness.[54]

The manifestations of symptomatic acute phase Chagas disease spontaneously resolve within 1 to 2 months, and the disease transitions into its chronic phase. Chronic Chagas disease is a lifelong infection; however, 60% to 70% of the infected individuals never develop clinically apparent sequalae and are considered to have an indeterminate form of the disease. Conversely, approximately one-third of infected patients experience a latency period of 10 to 30 years, after which they evolve to the determinate form of the chronic phase of Chagas disease, manifesting myriad cardiac, gastrointestinal (GI), and neurologic findings.[3]

Chagasic heart disease is the most common and serious manifestation of chronic T cruzi infection.[55] Conduction system abnormalities, particularly right bundle branch block and left anterior hemiblock, are the earliest signs of cardiac involvement.[56] As the disease progresses, patients develop atrial and ventricular arrhythmias, left ventricular dysfunction, thromboembolic events, dilated cardiomyopathy, and progressive congestive heart failure.[55–57] Consequently, patients manifest palpitations, syncope, and atypical chest pain.[56,57] In addition, there is a high risk of sudden death.[57] In fact, cardiac complications are the most common cause of Chagas-related mortality and account for approximately 21,000 deaths annually.[55] The most important prognostic predictors of chagasic heart disease are left ventricular dysfunction, heart failure that meets New York Heart Association functional class III/IV criteria, and presence of nonsustained ventricular tachycardia. Patients with these findings are deemed to be at highest risk for death and should, therefore, be managed aggressively.[55]

GI complications in chronic Chagas disease result from damage to intramural neurons with a direct affect on GI motility. Consequently, patients often experience dysphagia, esophageal reflux, aspiration, abdominal pain, constipation, and weight loss, with the most serious manifestations being megacolon and megaesophagus.[57,58]

While denervation of parasympathetic nerve fibers is largely responsible for the cardiac and GI manifestations of chronic Chagas disease, primary neurologic complications also occur. The most common findings are altered tendon reflexes and sensorimotor polyneuritis.[59] In addition, stroke secondary to cardioembolic events may represent the first presentation in chronic disease.[60]

Reactivation of Chagas disease may be observed in immunocompromised individuals, such as those with human immunodeficiency virus infection (HIV) or organ and bone marrow transplants. Although reactivated disease results in easily detectable parasitemia, the clinical presentation differs from that of acute Chagas disease and also differs between those with AIDS and transplant recipients.[57] Specifically, reactivation of Chagas disease in individuals coinfected with HIV is more likely to present with meningoencephalitis and space-occupying brain lesions.[57,61,62] By contrast, patients with reactivated disease who undergo transplant are more likely to develop cutaneous lesions of varying morphology including cellulitic plaques, inflammatory indurated nodules and plaques (**Fig. 1**), ulcers, necrotic eschars, and panniculitis (**Fig. 2**).[57,63–68] In both situations, patients with reactivation are often febrile, acutely ill, and may develop myocarditis.[57]

Diagnosis and Evaluation

Because of the resultant parasitemia during the acute phase of the illness, diagnosis of Chagas disease is made by microscopy, with identification of trymastigotes on peripheral blood smear. However, declining parasitemia in the chronic phase of the disease makes disease detection by microscopy unlikely. Consequently, diagnosis of chronic Chagas disease must be made by confirming the presence of anti–T cruzi IgG antibodies with at least 2 separate serologic tests such as enzyme-linked immunosorbent assay (ELISA), indirect hemagglutination, or indirect immunofluorescence. None of these tests have adequate sensitivity or specificity to be used alone; therefore 2 different methods must be used to sufficiently increase the accuracy of diagnosis. In addition,

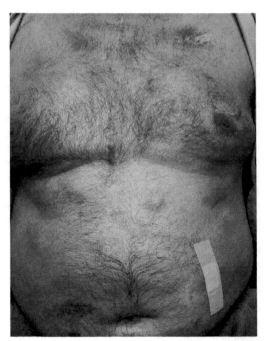

Fig. 1. Nodules and plaques in reactivated Chagas disease in a patient who has undergone transplant.

polymerase chain reaction (PCR)-based methods can provide a definitive diagnosis of Chagas disease during the acute phase of illness, but like microscopy, these methods are limited by the degree of parasitemia and are primarily used for research purposes only.[57]

In cases of suspected transplacental transmission, maternal diagnosis is established by the aforementioned serologic testing methods. To investigate congenital infection, infants born to seropositive mothers should be tested within the first 2 months of life via microscopic examination or PCR testing of cord and/or peripheral

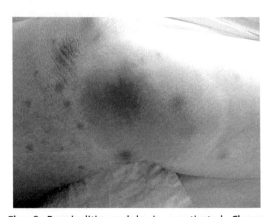

Fig. 2. Panniculitic nodule in reactivated Chagas disease.

blood.[57,69] If the results of initial testing are negative, follow-up serologic testing is recommended between the ages of 9 and 12 months.[57]

In the United States, 2 detection methods for use as screening tools are approved by the Food and Drug Administration. The first is the ORTHO *T cruzi* ELISA Test System (Ortho-Clinical Diagnostics Inc, Raritan, NJ, USA) approved in December 2006.[70] Subsequently, a second testing method was approved in April 2010, the ABBOTT PRISM Chagas chemiluminescent immunoassay (Abbott Laboratories, Abbott Park, IL, USA).[71] Both assays are used for qualitative antibody detection in serum and plasma specimens from whole blood, organ, cell, and tissue donors. Neither test is approved for diagnostic purposes.[70,71]

For seropositive individuals, the initial evaluation should consist of a thorough medical history, review of systems, and physical examination along with a 12-lead resting ECG. For asymptomatic patients with normal findings on ECG, the prognosis is good and yearly reevaluation is advised.[57]

For individuals with abnormalities in ECG or symptomatic disease, subsequent evaluation should be directed by that patient's specific symptoms or physical examination findings. For example, those with abnormalities in ECG or cardiac complaints should undergo a comprehensive cardiac workup to include 24-hour Holter monitoring, echocardiography, and exercise testing. The findings from these tests dictate the need for additional studies.[57]

For suspected GI involvement, patient should be evaluated by barium swallow and/or with enema. If testing is inconclusive, further studies may be indicated.[57]

In patients with cutaneous lesions, particularly in the setting of Chagas disease reactivation, diagnosis is often possible by skin biopsy. Histologic examination typically reveals a dense lymphohistiocytic infiltrate in the dermis and subcutis, along with numerous intracellular *T cruzi* amastigotes (**Fig. 3**), which display prominent kinetoplasts (**Fig. 4**) and are located within dermal macrophages.[21,63–66,68]

TREATMENT

Antiparasitic treatment is indicated for all cases of acute, congenital, and reactivated Chagas disease. The decision to treat chronic Chagas disease still remains somewhat controversial.[72,73] All children 18 years and younger with chronic Chagas disease should receive treatment. In adults aged 19 to 50 years without advanced cardiac involvement, antiparasitic therapy should

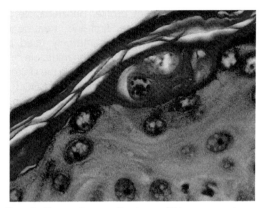

Fig. 3. *T cruzi* amastigotes within macrophages (Hematoxylin and eosin, original magnification ×40).

be offered and strongly considered. In patients older than 50 years, the risk of drug toxicity must be weighed against the benefits of treatment on an individual basis.[3,57,72,74]

However, of great importance in making this decision is the consideration of a study by Viotti and colleagues,[75] which demonstrated that antiparasitic agents may slow the progression of or even prevent cardiomyopathy in adults. For individuals with advanced cardiomyopathy, therapy with antiparasitic drugs is not recommended because treatment will not reverse the existing cardiac disease.[57] In addition, antitrypanosomal drugs are contraindicated in patients with advanced renal or hepatic disease and during pregnancy and breastfeeding.[3,57,72]

Only 2 medications have proven efficacy in the treatment of Chagas disease: benznidazole and nifurtimox. Because of its shorter treatment course

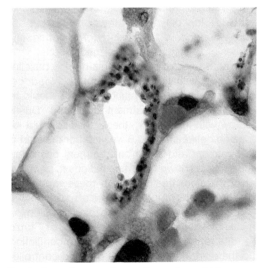

Fig. 4. Note the prominent kinetoplast within macrophages in a skin biopsy (Hematoxylin and eosin, original magnification ×100 [oil immersion]).

and superior side effect profile, benznidazole is generally considered the first-line treatment. However, nifurtimox is also commonly used in patients who do not tolerate benznidazole.[3,57] While neither drug is approved for use in the United States, both can be obtained through the CDC.[72]

Benznidazole, 5 to 7 mg/kg/d, is administered in 2 divided doses for 60 days. The most common adverse effects are cutaneous eruptions and peripheral neuropathy, both of which may occur in up to 30% of individuals treated. The associated cutaneous eruption that develops approximately 10 days after drug initiation is photosensitive pruritic dermatitis that can be managed symptomatically with topical corticosteroids. However, severe reactions including hypersensitivity syndromes with fever, lymphadenopathy, and exfoliative dermatitis have been reported and require prompt discontinuation of the drug. While benznidazole-induced neuropathy is dose-dependent, has a late onset, and is reversible, its development should also prompt discontinuation of the medication. Although bone marrow suppression is rare, monitoring of complete blood cell counts is mandated every 2 to 3 weeks. Less serious complaints associated with benznidazole therapy include anorexia, dysgeusia, nausea, vomiting, weight loss, and insomnia. It is important that patients taking benznidazole avoid alcohol consumption because of a disulfiram-like reaction.[57]

Nifurtimox, 8 to 10 mg/kg/d, is administered in 3 divided doses for 90 days. GI side effects are the most common and occur in a large number of patients treated with nifurtimox, including anorexia, weight loss, nausea, vomiting, and abdominal pain. In addition, individuals may experience vertigo, mood changes, and myalgia. Like benznidazole, polyneuropathy may occur as a dose-dependant late-onset complication and requires discontinuation of the medication.[57]

For both benznidazole and nifurtimox, baseline laboratory evaluation with complete blood cell count and liver and renal function tests should be performed before treatment initiation. During therapy with nifurtimox, these tests should be repeated between 4 and 6 weeks after the start of the treatment and again on treatment cessation. Studies have shown both medications to be mutagenic; therefore treatment with these drugs may potentially confer an increased risk of malignancy.[57]

Although allopurinol, itraconazole, and clomipramine have demonstrated efficacy against T cruzi, the data reported in the literature are conflicting, and there are no double-blind placebo-controlled trials to compare these agents against benznidazole or nifurtimox.[66,76–80] On the horizon are several molecules now under investigation as potential new drug targets for the treatment of Chagas disease, including both plant-based compounds with antitrypanosomal activity as well as proteins targets integral to T cruzi biochemical pathways.[81–84]

For patients with advanced chagasic heart disease, the use of pacemakers and implantable cardioverter defibrillators provide effective protection from arrhythmias and sudden cardiac death.[85,86] In addition, patients with end-stage dilated cardiomyopathy may be considered as candidates for heart transplant and have actually demonstrated superior survival rates than those receiving heart transplants for non-Chagas–related conditions.[87]

GI disease is often managed symptomatically with the goal of aiding swallowing and reducing constipation and fecal impaction. For cases that progress to megaesophagus or megacolon, surgical intervention may be necessary.[3]

Prevention and Control

The following general guidelines from the WHO are recommended for the control and prevention of Chagas disease: (1) applying insecticides in and around houses, (2) improving homes to reduce triatomine infestations, (3) using bed nets, (4) preparing and storing food properly, (5) screening all blood and tissue donors, and (6) screening neonates and their siblings born to infected mothers.[1]

As a result of a coordinated multination initiative in the Southern Cone nations of South America, the number of new Chagas infections has been reduced by 70%. This reduction has been achieved by directly interrupting both vector-borne and transfusional transmission of T cruzi through chemical control efforts, housing improvements, education, and blood donor screening. Because of the success of this initiative, similar programs are now being developed and implemented throughout many regions of Latin America. Consequently, the continued success of these programs will ultimately dictate a significant change in the current epidemiology of Chagas disease, with greater emphasis placed on transmission in nonendemic areas.[88]

In the last 5 years, considerable advances have been made toward the development of a Chagas disease vaccine, including the identification of major antigen targets, providing promise that a vaccine may soon become a reality.[89,90]

DISCUSSION

The impact of infection with T cruzi is steadily increasing in nonendemic regions such as the

United States and Europe, largely because of globalization of travel and immigration patterns that have brought about major shifts in the epidemiology of Chagas disease.[14,16,27,91] In addition, the emergence of AIDS as a worldwide epidemic and the increasing prevalence of organ and bone marrow transplants have further altered the epidemiology of this disease by providing new avenues for disease transmission and reactivation. Thus, the emergence of Chagas disease as a public health concern demands increased awareness from physicians in the United States, Canada, and Europe.[14,27,43,44,91,92] In fact, some investigators think that several chagasic heart disease cases are being misdiagnosed as dilated idiopathic cardiomyopathy. The recognition that Chagas disease now represents a true threat in nonendemic regions should spur clinicians to have an increased index of suspicion for this diagnosis.[93] Furthermore, it is argued that to successfully combat this disease in the future, nonendemic nations must now join the effort to resolve the limitations of the understanding of the pathogenesis of Chagas disease and pursue new molecular targets for vaccines and drug therapies.[84]

REFERENCES

1. Chagas disease (American trypanosomiasis) Fact Sheet No. 340. World Health Organization website. Available at: http://www.who.int/mediacentre/factsheets/fs340/en/index.html. Accessed August 7, 2010.

2. Araújo A, Jansen AM, Reinhard K, et al. Paleoparasitology of Chagas disease—a review. Mem Inst Oswaldo Cruz 2009;104(Suppl 1):9–16.

3. Rassi A Jr, Rassi A, Marin-Neto JA. Chagas disease. Lancet 2010;375:1388–402.

4. Chagas disease—Detailed FAQs. Centers for Disease Control and Prevention website. Available at: http://www.cdc.gov/chagas/gen_info/detailed.html. Accessed August 7, 2010.

5. Centers for Disease Control and Prevention. Blood donor screening for Chagas disease—United States, 2006–2007. MMWR Morb Mortal Wkly Rep 2007;56(7):141–3.

6. Leiby DA, Herron RM Jr, Garratty G, et al. *Trypanosoma cruzi* parasitemia in US blood donors with serologic evidence of infection. J Infect Dis 2008;198(4):609–13.

7. Bern C, Montgomery SP, Katz L, et al. Chagas disease and the US blood supply. Curr Opin Infect Dis 2008;21(5):476–82.

8. Centers for Disease Control and Prevention. Chagas disease after organ transplantation—United States, 2001. MMWR Morb Mortal Wkly Rep 2002;51(10):210–2.

9. Centers for Disease Control and Prevention. Chagas disease after organ transplantation—Los Angeles, California, 2006. MMWR Morb Mortal Wkly Rep 2006;55(29):798–800.

10. Bryan CF, Tegtmeier GE, Rafik N, et al. The risk for Chagas' disease in the Midwestern United States organ donor population is low. Clin Transplant 2004;18(12):12–5.

11. Nowicki MJ, Chinchilla C, Corado L, et al. Prevalence of antibodies to *Trypanosoma cruzi* among solid organ donors in Southern California: a population at risk. Transplantation 2006;81(3):477–9.

12. Pérez-López FR, Chedraui P. Chagas disease in pregnancy: a non-endemic problem in a globalized world. Arch Gynecol Obstet 2010. [Epub ahead of print].

13. Herwaldt BL. Laboratory-acquired parasitic infections from accidental exposures. Clin Microbiol Rev 2001;14(4):659–88.

14. Schmunis GA. Epidemiology of Chagas disease in non-endemic countries: the role of international migration. Mem Inst Oswaldo Cruz 2007;102(Suppl 1):75–85.

15. Migration and the movement of infectious diseases: Chagas disease. Centers for Disease Control and Prevention website. Available at: http://www.cdc.gov/nczved/framework/features/chagas.html. Accessed August 7, 2010.

16. Kirchhoff LV. American trypanosomiasis (Chagas' disease)—a tropical disease now in the United States. N Engl J Med 1993;329:639–44.

17. Altclas J, Jaimovich G, Milovic V, et al. Chagas' disease after bone marrow transplantation. Bone Marrow Transplant 1996;18(2):447–8.

18. Villalba R, Fornés G, Alvarez MA, et al. Acute Chagas' disease in a recipient of a bone marrow transplant in Spain: case report. Clin Infect Dis 1992;14(2):594–5.

19. Machado CM, Martins TC, Colturato I, et al. Epidemiology of neglected tropical diseases in transplant recipients. Review of the literature and experience of a Brazilian HSCT center. Rev Inst Med Trop Sao Paulo 2009;51(6):309–24.

20. Chocair PR, Sabbaga E, Amato Neto V, et al. Kidney transplantation: a new way of transmitting Chagas disease. Rev Inst Med Trop Sao Paulo 1981;23:280–2.

21. Riarte A, Luna C, Sabatiello R, et al. Chagas' disease in patients with kidney transplants: 7 years of experience 1989–1996. Clin Infect Dis 1999;29(3):561–7.

22. Jackson Y, Myers C, Diana A, et al. Congenital transmission of Chagas disease in Latin American immigrants in Switzerland. Emerg Infect Dis 2009;15(4):601–3.

23. Pereira KS, Schmidt FL, Barbosa RL, et al. Transmission of Chagas disease (American trypanosomiasis) by food. Adv Food Nutr Res 2010;59C:63–85.

24. Nóbrega AA, Garcia MH, Tatto E, et al. Oral transmission of Chagas disease by consumption of açaí palm fruit, Brazil. Emerg Infect Dis 2009;15(4): 653–5.

25. Alarcón de Noya B, Díaz-Bello Z, Colmenares C, et al. Large urban outbreak of orally acquired acute Chagas disease at a school in Caracas, Venezuela. J Infect Dis 2010;201(9):1308–15.

26. Chagas disease epidemiology & risk factors. Centers for Disease Control and Prevention website. Available at: http://www.cdc.gov/chagas/epi.html. Accessed August 7, 2010.

27. Dorn P, Buekens P, Hanford E. Whac-a-mole: future trends in Chagas transmission and the importance of a global perspective on disease control. Future Microbiol 2007;2:365–7.

28. Viotti R, Vigliano CA, Alvarez MG, et al. The impact of socioeconomic conditions on chronic Chagas disease progression. Rev Esp Cardiol 2009;62(11): 1224–32.

29. Control of neglected tropical diseases. World Health Organization website. Available at: http://www.who.int/neglected_diseases/en/index.html. Accessed August 7, 2010.

30. Epidemiological profiles of neglected diseases and other infections related to poverty in Latin America and the Caribbean. Pan American Health Organization website. Available at: http://new.paho.org/hq/index.php?option=com_joomlabook&Itemid=259&task=display&id=58. Accessed August 7, 2010.

31. Strosberg AM, Barrio K, Stinger VH, et al. Chagas disease: a Latin American nemesis. 2007. Institute for OneWorld Health website. Available at: http://www.oneworldhealth.org/documents/CHAGAS%20Landscape%20FINAL%20VERSION.pdf. Accessed August 7, 2010.

32. Chagas disease in the Americas: no longer exotic 2009 fact sheet. Centers for Disease Control and Prevention website. Available at: http://www.cdc.gov/chagas/resources/chagas_no_longer_an_exotic_disease.pdf. Accessed August 7, 2010.

33. Herwaldt BL, Grijalva MJ, Newsome AL, et al. Use of polymerase chain reaction to diagnose the fifth reported U.S. case of autochthonous transmission of Trypanosoma cruzi—Tennessee, 1998. J Infect Dis 2000;181:395–9.

34. Reisenman CE, Lawrence G, Guerenstein PG, et al. Infection of kissing bugs with Trypanosoma cruzi, Tucson, Arizona, USA. Emerg Infect Dis 2010; 16(3):400–5.

35. Barr SC, Brown CC, Dennis VA, et al. The lesions and prevalence of Trypanosoma cruzi in opossums and armadillos from southern Louisiana. J Parasitol 1991;77:624–7.

36. Yabsley MJ, Noblet GP. Seroprevalence of Trypanosoma cruzi in raccoons from South Carolina and Georgia. J Wildl Dis 2002;38(1):75–83.

37. Barr SC, Dennis VA, Klei TR. Serological and blood culture survey of Trypanosoma cruzi infection in four canine populations of southern Louisiana. Am J Vet Res 1991;52:570–3.

38. Barr SC, Gossett KA, Klei TR. Clinical, clinicopathologic, and parasitologic observations of trypanosomiasis in dogs infected with North American Trypanosoma cruzi isolates. Am J Vet Res 1991;52: 954–60.

39. Burkholder JE, Allison TC, Kelly VP, et al. Chronic Trypanosoma cruzi infection in dogs: 11 cases (1987–1996). J Am Vet Med Assoc 1998;213: 497–500.

40. Beard CB, Pye G, Steurer FJ, et al. Chagas disease in a domestic transmission cycle, southern Texas, USA. Emerg Infect Dis 2003;9(1):103–5.

41. Kjos SA, Snowden KF, Craig TM, et al. Distribution and characterization of canine Chagas disease in Texas. Vet Parasitol 2008;152(3–4):249–56.

42. Rowland ME, Maloney J, Cohen S, et al. Factors associated with Trypanosoma cruzi exposure among domestic canines in Tennessee. J Parasitol 2010;96(3):547–51.

43. Diaz JH. Chagas disease in the United States: a cause for concern in Louisiana? J La State Med Soc 2007;159(1):21–3, 25–9.

44. Hanford EJ, Zhan FB, Lu Y, et al. Chagas disease in Texas: recognizing the significance and implications of evidence in the literature. Soc Sci Med 2007; 65(1):60–79.

45. Noireau F, Diosque P, Jansen AM. Trypanosoma cruzi: adaptation to its vectors and its hosts. Vet Res 2009; 40(2):26–8.

46. Dutra WO, Gollob KJ. Current concepts in immunoregulation and pathology of human Chagas disease. Curr Opin Infect Dis 2008;21(3):287–92.

47. Scharfstein J, Gomes Jde A, Correa-Oliveira R. Back to the future in Chagas disease: from animal models to patient cohort studies, progress in immunopathogenesis research. Mem Inst Oswaldo Cruz 2009;104(Suppl 1):187–98.

48. Teixeira AR, Nitz N, Guimaro MC, et al. Chagas disease. Postgrad Med J 2006;82(974):788–98.

49. Gironès N, Cuervo H, Fresno M. Trypanosoma cruzi-induced molecular mimicry and Chagas' disease. Curr Top Microbiol Immunol 2005;296:89–123.

50. Piacenza L, Alvarez MN, Peluffo G, et al. Fighting the oxidative assault: the Trypanosoma cruzi journey to infection. Curr Opin Microbiol 2009;12(4):415–21.

51. Villalta F, Scharfstein J, Ashton AW, et al. Perspectives on the Trypanosoma cruzi-host cell receptor interactions. Parasitol Res 2009;104(6):1251–60.

52. Padilla AM, Bustamante JM, Tarleton RL. CD8+ T cells in Trypanosoma cruzi infection. Curr Opin Immunol 2009;21(4):385–90.

53. Gutierrez FR, Mineo TW, Pavanelli WR, et al. The effects of nitric oxide on the immune system during

Trypanosoma cruzi infection. Mem Inst Oswaldo Cruz 2009;104(Suppl 1):236–45.

54. Lupi O, Bartlett BL, Haugen RN, et al. Tropical dermatology: tropical diseases caused by protozoa. J Am Acad Dermatol 2009;60:897–925.

55. Rassi A Jr, Rassi A, Rassi SG. Predictors of mortality in chronic Chagas disease: a systematic review of observational studies. Circulation 2007;115(9):1101–8.

56. Blum JA, Zellweger MJ, Burri C, et al. Cardiac involvement in African and American trypanosomiasis. Lancet Infect Dis 2008;8(10):631–41.

57. Bern C, Montgomery SP, Herwaldt BL, et al. Evaluation and treatment of Chagas disease in the United States: a systematic review. JAMA 2007;298(18):2171–81.

58. Matsuda NM, Miller SM, Evora PR. The chronic gastrointestinal manifestations of Chagas disease. Clinics (Sao Paulo) 2009;64(12):1219–24.

59. Córdova E, Maiolo E, Corti M, et al. Neurological manifestations of Chagas' disease. Neurol Res 2010;32(3):238–44.

60. Carod-Artal FJ, Gascon J. Chagas disease and stroke. Lancet Neurol 2010;9(5):533–42.

61. Ferreira MS, Nishioka Sde A, Silvestre MT, et al. Reactivation of Chagas' disease in patients with AIDS: report of three new cases and review of the literature. Clin Infect Dis 1997;25(6):1397–400.

62. Diazgranados CA, Saavedra-Trujillo CH, Mantilla M, et al. Chagasic encephalitis in HIV patients: common presentation of an evolving epidemiological and clinical association. Lancet Infect Dis 2009;9(5):324–30.

63. Gallerano V, Consigli J, Pereyra S, et al. Chagas' disease reactivation with skin symptoms in a patient with kidney transplant. Int J Dermatol 2007;46(6):607–10.

64. Hall CS, Fields K. Cutaneous presentation of Chagas' disease reactivation in a heart-transplant patient in Utah. J Am Acad Dermatol 2008;58(3):529–30.

65. La Forgia MP, Pellerano G, de las Mercedes Portaluppi M, et al. Cutaneous manifestation of reactivation of Chagas disease in a renal transplant patient: long-term follow-up. Arch Dermatol 2003;139(1):104–5.

66. Tomimori-Yamashita J, Deps PD, Almeida DR, et al. Cutaneous manifestation of Chagas' disease after heart transplantation: successful treatment with allopurinol. Br J Dermatol 1997;137(4):626–30.

67. Amato JG, Amato Neto V, Amato VS, et al. Cutaneous lesions as the only manifestations of reactions to *Trypanosoma cruzi* infection in a recipient of a kidney transplant. Rev Soc Bras Med Trop 1996;30(1):61–3.

68. Libow LF, Beltrani VP, Silvers DN, et al. Post-cardiac transplant reactivation of Chagas' disease diagnosed by skin biopsy. Cutis 1991;48(1):37–40.

69. Mora MC, Sanchez Negrette O, Marco D, et al. Early diagnosis of congenital *Trypanosoma cruzi* infection using PCR, hemoculture, and capillary concentration, as compared with delayed serology. J Parasitol 2005;91(6):1468–73.

70. ORTHO *T. cruzi* ELISA Test System. U.S. Food and Drug Administration website. Available at: http://www.fda.gov/BiologicsBloodVaccines/BloodBloodProducts/ApprovedProducts/LicensedProductsBLAs/BloodDonorScreening/InfectiousDisease/ucm085846.htm. Accessed August 7, 2010.

71. Abbott prism Chagas. U.S. Food and Drug Administration website. Available at: http://www.fda.gov/BiologicsBloodVaccines/BloodBloodProducts/ApprovedProducts/LicensedProductsBLAs/BloodDonorScreening/InfectiousDisease/ucm210158.htm. Accessed August 7, 2010.

72. Chagas disease–antiparasitic treatment. Centers for Disease Control and Prevention website. Available at: http://www.cdc.gov/chagas/health_professionals/tx.html. Accessed August 7, 2010.

73. Reyes PA, Vallejo M. Trypanocidal drugs for late stage, symptomatic Chagas disease (*Trypanosoma cruzi* infection). Cochrane Database Syst Rev 2005;4:CD004102.

74. Pérez-Molina JA, Pérez-Ayala A, Moreno S, et al. Use of benznidazole to treat chronic Chagas' disease: a systematic review with a meta-analysis. J Antimicrob Chemother 2009;64(6):1139–47.

75. Viotti R, Vigliano C, Lococo B, et al. Long-term cardiac outcomes of treating chronic Chagas disease with benznidazole versus no treatment: a nonrandomized trial. Ann Intern Med 2006;144(10):724–34.

76. Gobbi P, Baez A, Lo Presti MS, et al. Association of clomipramine and allopurinol for the treatment of the experimental infection with *Trypanosoma cruzi*. Parasitol Res 2010;107(5):127–83.

77. Gobbi P, Lo Presti MS, Fernández AR, et al. Allopurinol is effective to modify the evolution of *Trypanosoma cruzi* infection in mice. Parasitol Res 2007;101(5):1459–62.

78. Rassi A, Luquetti AO, Rassi A Jr, et al. Specific treatment for *Trypanosoma cruzi*: lack of efficacy of allopurinol in the human chronic phase of Chagas disease. Am J Trop Med Hyg 2007;76(1):58–61.

79. Apt W, Arribada A, Zulantay I, et al. Itraconazole or allopurinol in the treatment of chronic American trypanosomiasis: the results of clinical and parasitological examinations 11 years post-treatment. Ann Trop Med Parasitol 2005;99(8):733–41.

80. Almeida DR, Carvalho AC, Branco JN, et al. Chagas' disease reactivation after heart transplantation: efficacy of allopurinol treatment. J Heart Lung Transplant 1996;15(10):988–92.

81. Pinto AV, de Castro SL. The trypanocidal activity of naphthoquinones: a review. Molecules 2009;14(11):4570–90.

82. Sánchez-Sancho F, Campillo NE, Páez JA. Chagas disease: progress and new perspectives. Curr Med Chem 2010;17(5):423–52.

83. Rivera G, Bocanegra-García V, Ordaz-Pichardo C, et al. New therapeutic targets for drug design against *Trypanosoma cruzi*, advances and perspectives. Curr Med Chem 2009;16(25): 3286–93.

84. Ribeiro I, Sevcsik AM, Alves F, et al. New, improved treatments for Chagas disease: from the R&D pipeline to the patients. PLoS Negl Trop Dis 2009;3(7): e484.

85. Muratore CA, Batista Sa LA, Chiale PA, et al. Implantable cardioverter defibrillators and Chagas' disease: results of the ICD registry Latin America. Europace 2009;11(2):164–8.

86. Dubner S, Schapachnik E, Riera AR, et al. Chagas disease: state-of-the-art of diagnosis and management. Cardiol J 2008;15(6):493–504.

87. Bestetti RB, Theodoropoulos TA. A systematic review of studies on heart transplantation for patients with end-stage Chagas' heart disease. J Card Fail 2009;15(3):249–55.

88. Moncayo A. Chagas disease: current epidemiological trends after the interruption of vectorial and transfusional transmission in the Southern Cone countries. Mem Inst Oswaldo Cruz 2003;98(5): 577–91.

89. Cazorla SI, Frank FM, Malchiodi EL. Vaccination approaches against *Trypanosoma cruzi* infection. Expert Rev Vaccines 2009;8(7):921–35.

90. Duschak VG, Couto AS. Cruzipain, the major cysteine protease of *Trypanosoma cruzi*: a sulfated glycoprotein antigen as relevant candidate for vaccine development and drug target. A review. Curr Med Chem 2009;16(24):3174–202.

91. Milei J, Guerri-Guttenberg RA, Grana DR, et al. Prognostic impact of Chagas disease in the United States. Am Heart J 2009;157(1):22–9.

92. Guerri-Guttenberg RA, Grana DR, Ambrosio G, et al. Chagas cardiomyopathy: Europe is not spared! Eur Heart J 2008;29(21):2587–91.

93. Milei J, Mautner B, Storino R, et al. Does Chagas' disease exist as an undiagnosed form of cardiomyopathy in the United States? Am Heart J 1992; 123(6):1732–5.

Dermatology in Botswana: The American Academy of Dermatology's Resident International Grant

Camille E. Introcaso, MD[a,b], Carrie L. Kovarik, MD[c,d],*

KEYWORDS

- International dermatology • Volunteerism • Teledermatology
- Tropical dermatology • Dermatology education

"Dumela, Ma!" Across the globe, a North American dermatology resident greets a patient at the skin clinic at Princess Marina Hospital in Gaborone, Botswana. The patient has waited that morning with as many as 30 other patients to see the resident, who is one of only two dermatologists working in the country's public health sector. The resident conducts the interview and examination with the assistance of a nurse who speaks English and Tswana (Setswana), the language spoken by many in Botswana. The resident makes a diagnosis, discusses the plan of care with the patient, and writes a brief note and prescription in the chart the patient carries with her; the patient heads to the hospital pharmacy. Later that afternoon, the resident does inpatient consultations, discusses management with the teams of local doctors and nurses, and makes plans to give a lecture and see patients at a neighboring rural clinic the following week. At the end of the day, the resident returns to the Botswana-UPenn Partnership-owned flat with medical students and residents from North America, and the group shares dinner and the various experiences they have had that day conducting research in the clinics and on the inpatient wards.

The American Academy of Dermatology (AAD) has a long tradition of volunteerism. From its involvement with Camp Discovery to the multitude of AAD-supported skin cancer screenings and the monthly highlight of "Members Making a Difference" in its newsletter, the Academy has consistently provided its members with encouragement and opportunities to use their skills to reach vulnerable or underserved communities. Over the last 3 years, a group of motivated AAD members and educators have linked together a network of domestic and international health organizations to create a unique opportunity for dermatology residents to further their education and provide care to a sub-Saharan African population. This article highlights the history, elements, and scope

This work discusses a project supported by the American Academy of Dermatology.
The authors have no conflicts of interest to disclose.
a Department of Dermatology, Pennsylvania Hospital, 800 Spruce Street, Philadelphia, PA 19107, USA
b Pennsylvania Center for Dermatology, 801 Spruce Street, Philadelphia, PA 19107, USA
c Department of Dermatology , Hospital of the University of Pennsylvania, 3600 Spruce Street, Philadelphia, PA 19104, USA
d Division of Infectious Disease, Department of Internal Medicine, Hospital of the University of Pennsylvania, Philadelphia, PA 19104, USA
* Corresponding author. Department of Dermatology, Hospital of the University of Pennsylvania, 3600 Spruce Street, Philadelphia, PA 19104.
E-mail address: Carrie.kovarik@uphs.upenn.edu

Dermatol Clin 29 (2011) 63–67
doi:10.1016/j.det.2010.09.001

of the program called the Resident International Grant.

HISTORY OF THE RESIDENT'S INTERNATIONAL GRANT

In 2008, the Education and Volunteers Abroad Committee of the AAD approached the AAD leadership and requested support and funding to send six residents to live and work in Gaborone, Botswana, and the Resident International Grant was created. Three main partnerships had been forged, providing housing, in-country support, and connection to health care services in Botswana needed by the dermatology residents. In the early 2000s, the Infectious Disease Division of the Hospital of the University of Pennsylvania (UPenn) established a relationship with the Ministry of Health and Princess Marina Hospital in Botswana. Since then, UPenn medical students and residents had lived in the community in shared flats in Gaborone and rotated through the adult inpatient wards of Princess Marina Hospital. Similarly, the Baylor International Pediatrics AIDS Initiative (BIPAI) had developed a partnership with Princess Marina Hospital, providing education, staffing, and funding for an outpatient pediatrics clinic for the care of pediatric HIV patients. These academic institutions were linked by a group of dermatologists with shared experiences with both, in particular Dr Carrie Kovarik, who would later become the director of the Resident International Grant. Through funding provided by the Association of Professors of Dermatology in 2007, the first two formally-supported dermatology residents traveled to Botswana and worked with the one existing dermatologist in the public sector.

From these early experiences, it became clear that both the patients of Botswana and the North American dermatology residents could benefit from the residents' presence at Princess Marina Hospital. The residents would receive the invaluable experiences of seeing and treating tropical and HIV-associated dermatoses and have the opportunity to learn to provide general dermatologic care and education to a different culture in a resource-limited setting. The patients would be provided with additional well-trained dermatologists, and the health care workers of Botswana would be provided with further education on dermatologic disease to build their capacity for future care. With these opportunities in mind and the instrumental support of Dr William James, the current President of the AAD, the Academy approved the initial positions. The responses of the residents who completed the program, the leadership of the organizations involved, and the

patients were so positive that additional positions were and continue to be approved for virtually continuous coverage of the clinic through to the end of 2011.

"YOU'RE GOING WHERE?" AN INTRODUCTION TO BOTSWANA

Botswana is a landlocked country in sub-Saharan Africa. The population of Botswana is approximately 2 million, with most people living in the southwest corner of the country. Most of central Botswana consists of the largely uninhabitable Kalahari desert. The country is best known for tourism and has thriving safari parks in the north. Its economy is otherwise based on diamond mining and cattle herding. Since its independence from Great Britain in 1966, Botswana has been a democratic republic, and it has enjoyed a long history of peace and relative prosperity compared with the civil unrest experienced by some of its neighbors. However, in the 1990s, it became apparent that the people of Botswana were being disproportionately affected by the HIV epidemic; by 2006, it was estimated that 26% of the adult population was HIV-positive.[1] Parallel private and government-funded public systems comprise the health care system in Botswana, with most of the country dependent on the public system. In the early 2000s, the public health care system began a comprehensive HIV care program that included antiretroviral treatment, bringing many living with HIV into the health care system. HIV-related dermatoses are heavily represented in the diagnoses made in the dermatology clinic where the residents work. Despite its relative stability, a large proportion of Botswana's population is poor, and the public health care sector is stretched thin in some areas. Access to specialty care, including dermatologic care, is very limited in the public sector, and many patients seen at the Princess Marina Skin Clinic have traveled great distances.

RESIDENT RESPONSIBILITIES

Residents who participate in the Resident International Grant spend four to six weeks living and working in Gaborone, Botswana. Approximately three days a week, 20 to 40 patients are scheduled in the outpatient "Skin Clinic" on the Princess Marina Hospital campus. The resident often sees patients independently but also works together with the other public sector dermatologist. Each weekday, the resident is responsible for seeing the clinic patients, working with the pathologist and microbiologist at the neighboring National

Laboratory to follow up on the clinic's pathology and laboratory results, and providing pediatric and adult inpatient consultations at Princess Marina Hospital. Residents are expected to keep a basic log and when appropriate photographic record of patients that they have seen. The common diagnoses include much of what is seen in a general dermatology clinic in North America, such as acne and atopic dermatitis, with an emphasis on photodermatoses, including discoid lupus and phototoxic and photoallergic medication reactions; pigmentation abnormalities; oculocutaneous albinism; and infectious disease, including superficial fungal and bacterial infections. Also seen are many manifestations of HIV, such as papular pruritic eruption, herpes virus infections, human papilloma virus infections, molluscum contagiosum, deep fungal infections, atypical mycobacterial infections, and Kaposi sarcoma (**Fig. 1**). The hospital pharmacy stocks a very basic formulary and medication is provided to the patients at low or no cost through the public health care program.

Capacity-building in the form of dermatology education to local health care workers is a crucial component of the program. Over the course of the rotation, the resident gives several didactic presentations to groups of health care providers associated with Princess Marina Hospital, surrounding district hospitals, the BIPAI, and/or community organizations. Often, other opportunities to teach arise; the community living situation lends itself to the development of friendships and collaborative relationships, and dermatology residents are often shadowed by medical students or other residents living with them. The University of Botswana internal medicine and pediatrics residents formally complete a one-month rotation on the dermatology service, and the dermatology resident has the opportunity for hands-on teaching, while learning more about general medicine in Botswana from the local physicians. About once a week, the resident has the opportunity to travel by bus, taxi, or with other health care workers to one of four neighboring clinics and hospitals in the rural areas outside Gaborone. At these clinics, the resident sees out- and inpatients and lectures on helpful dermatology topics to local care providers. A one-week overlap between the residents ensures continuity in the service and gives residents a chance to interact with and learn from their peers.

Although running the dermatology service fairly autonomously is a valuable part of the experience, several programs are in place to ensure that residents have sufficient support to provide excellent care. The residents work closely with the public sector dermatologist in Princess Marina Hospital, Dr Gilberto Lopez, a Cuban physician who is currently living and working in Botswana. Another service that provides support is teledermatology, and one of the goals of the Resident International Grant is to educate the residents in using teledermatology services effectively. The resident can submit consultations on an Internet-based store-and-forward system (http://africa.telederm.org) or by mobile (cellular) teledermatology; the resident is provided with a cellular phone equipped with a 5.0-megapixel camera and ClickDoc (Click Diagnostics, Boston, MA, USA) software, which allows for submission of cases without an Internet connection. The consultations are answered by a group of dermatologists organized by Dr Kovarik, who is always available for clinical or social support during

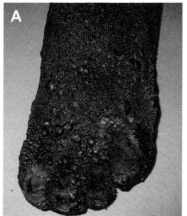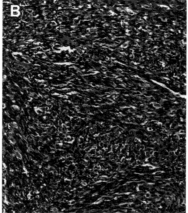

Fig. 1. (*A*) Clinical image of a patient at Princess Marina Skin Clinic with Kaposi sarcoma. (*B*) Photomicrograph taken using remote microscope. (*Courtesy of* Dr Saurabh Singh, MD, Washington, DC).

a resident's time in Botswana. The residents are expected to submit a certain number of teledermatology consultations during their rotation to provide high-quality care, get feedback on their diagnoses and management plans, and have enough experience with the technology to teach the next resident.

Histopathology interpretation support is another important component of the residents' experience. Dr Scott Binder at the University of California, Los Angeles (UCLA) Department of Pathology generously facilitated the donation of a live telepathology system (Zeiss Mirax Live RT system, Carl Zeiss Microlmaging GmbH, Jena, Germany) for interpretation of skin biopsies and teaching local pathologists in Botswana (see **Fig. 1**). Along with Dr Kovarik, members of the UCLA dermatopathology faculty regularly volunteer and provide interpretations of cutaneous histopathology to assist and educate the dermatology residents and the busy pathology department at the National Laboratory of Botswana. Generally residents work as a team with the local pathologist, Dr M Kayembe, to determine which slides to load on the microscope, and the team discusses the case with the consulting dermatopathologists through teledermatology.

As the program has evolved and become better defined, there have been several opportunities for residents to participate in and conduct clinical research while in Botswana. Residents have assisted with local clinical trials, with research on teledermatology and teledermatopathology services, with human-papillomavirus-related malignancies, and with various case reports based on their experiences.

SUMMARY

Following their return home, the residents are asked to write a reflection on their experiences for the program leadership at the AAD to identify strengths of the program and areas for improvement and growth. These reflections have been a valuable source of information and have been extremely positive about the depth and breadth of the residents' experiences. For many, this was their first experience as dermatologists in a foreign culture or working in a resource-limited setting, and most comment on their desire to continue similar work or volunteer activities. As a testament to the popularity of the program, the number of applications received for the 2011 grant rotation has nearly doubled since 2008.

Since the first residents traveled to Gaborone, Botswana in 2008, more than 1500 patients have been seen as part of the Resident International Grant. Dozens of teledermatology and teledermatopathology consultations have been sent and discussed, and almost 50 dermatology lectures have been given across Botswana. More than 50 residents have applied, and by the end of 2010, 35 residents will have traveled to Botswana and completed the rotation. Anyone interested in learning more about the program or applying for a future position is requested to visit the AAD Web site for more detailed information. As the Resident International Grant enters its fourth year, it seems clear that although much work remains to be done, there are many academy members and dermatology residents who are more than willing to undertake it. Finally, the supporters of the program hoped that the local clinicians gain the knowledge and hands-on experience to allow them to sustain dermatologic care for the patients in Botswana.

ACKNOWLEDGMENTS

The authors would like to thank the following people and organizations for making this possible: the AAD; Coura Badiane and the AAD Education and Volunteers Abroad Committee; William D James, MD; Michael Kramer, MD; the Botswana-UPenn Partnership; the UCLA Department of Pathology and Scott Binder, MD; the BIPAI; the Botswana Ministry of Health; the University of Botswana; the staff of Princess Marina Hospital; the Association of Professors of Dermatology (APD); Dr M Kayembe; Dr Gilberto Lopez; Robert Lee, MD, PhD; Juliette Lee, MD, Jing Gill, MD; Eunice Tsai, MD; Jeremy Kampp, MD; Max Fischer, MD, MPH; all the residents and faculty members that have participated in this program: Jackie Panko, MD, University of Utah; Jennifer Mueller, MD, Drexel University; Felisa Lewis, MD, National Capital Consortium Dermatology Program; Leslie Castelo-Socio, MD, PhD, UPenn; David Wartman, MD, Brown; Chris Jones, MD, Penn State Hershey; Rachael Moore, MD, Oregon Health Sciences University, Ivy Lee, MD, Georgetown University Hospital; Yvette Miller-Monthrope, MD, University of Toronto; Marissa Joseph, MD, University of Toronto; Quyn Sherrod, MD, UCLA; Emily Fridlington, MD, University of Iowa, Camille Introcaso MD, UPenn; Melanie Walter, MD, Duke University; Melinda Jen, MD, University of Connecticut; Ron Bernardin, MD, UPenn; Pristine Lee, MD, University of California San Diego; Alaina James, MD, PhD, UPenn; Rahat Azfar, MD, UPenn; David Carr, MD, Wright State University; Saurabh Singh, MD, Georgetown University Hospital; Shannon Campbell, DO, Ohio University/O'Bleness Memorial Hospital

Dermatology Residency Program; Jennifer Tan-Billet, MD, Harvard Combined Dermatology Residency; Paul Tumeh, MD, PhD, Harbor — UCLA Dermatology; Emma Taylor, MD, UCLA; Jennifer Gardner, MD, UPenn; Casey Carlos, MD, PhD, UPenn; Tace Rico, MD, University of Miami Dermatology; Nisha Mistry, MD, University of British Columbia; Nic Compton, MD, University of Washington; Sarah Rodgers, MD, Duke University; Anthony Rossi, MD, Cornell University.

REFERENCE

1. UNAIDS. Available at: http://www.unaids.org/en/KnowledgeCentre/HIVData/GlobalReport/2006/. Accessed June 24, 2010.

Effectiveness of Gentian Violet and Similar Products Commonly Used to Treat Pyodermas

Ricardo L. Berrios, MD[a],*, Jack L. Arbiser, MD, PhD[a,b]

KEYWORDS

- Pyoderma • Triphenylmethane • Gentian violet
- Vascular leak

Loosely defined as a bacterial infection of the skin, the term pyoderma encompasses a variety of distinct entities, including impetigo (bullous and nonbullous), erysipelas, cellulitis, folliculitis, and staphylococcal scalded skin syndrome. The pathogens responsible for these conditions are mainly gram-positive bacteria native to the skin flora (*Staphylococcus aureus* and *Streptococcus pyogenes*). Treatment of pyodermas centers around wound care and appropriate antibiotic selection, but in the age of increasing bacterial resistance (particularly methicillin-resistant *S aureus* [MRSA]) there is always an ongoing search for alternative and effective agents. Triphenylmethanes represent a unique group of compounds with a variety of properties including antisepsis (**Table 1**). This article reviews some applications of these compounds as they relate to pyodermas.

ALTERNATIVES IN THE FACE OF ANTIBIOTIC RESISTANCE

In the United States, an estimated 95 million people are nasal carriers of *S aureus*; of these, 2.6% or 2.5 million people carry the methicillin-resistant organism.[1] A study in 2004 found the incidence of community-acquired MRSA to be between 15% and 75% in 11 university-associated emergency departments.[2] Although not all acquisitions of MRSA are associated with the development of disease, it is imperative that when physicians encounter a skin and soft tissue infection, (SSTI) they should be aware of the rates of MRSA in their communities in addition to the risk factors present in each patient so that appropriate therapy may be initiated promptly. Risk factors for community-acquired MRSA include close physical contact, poor hygiene, shared sanitary facilities, and living in crowded conditions (eg, military recruits and prisons).[3]

Currently, oral agents used to treat MRSA-associated infections include clindamycin, trimethoprim-sulfamethoxazole, tetracyclines, and, less commonly, linezolid; topical mupirocin has also shown efficacy. Of these, a linezolid-resistant strain of MRSA has already been documented in a hospital setting in Spain.[4] As such, the search for effective and well-tolerated agents is ongoing; one commonly overlooked agent is gentian violet (GV). GV has a varied and lengthy history as a medicinal agent. Both bacteriostatic and bacteriocidal, GV's utility in antisepsis and thrush and as an antitreponemal agent are well documented[5–8]; its first mention in the literature dates back to 1912.[9] Hinton[10] administered GV intravenously to patients with severe sepsis and showed notable efficacy. Once quite commonplace, GV has since

[a] Department of Dermatology, Emory University School of Medicine, 101 Woodruff Circle, Suite 5339, Atlanta, GA 30322, USA
[b] Division of Dermatology, Atlanta Veterans Administration Medical Center, 1670 Clairmont Road, Decatur, GA 30033, USA
* Corresponding author.
E-mail address: rberrio@emory.edu

Dermatol Clin 29 (2011) 69–73
doi:10.1016/j.det.2010.08.009

Table 1
Examples of triphenylmethane dyes with accepted medical uses, dermatologic indications, and pertinent side effects

Compound	Structure	Medical Uses[25]	Dermatologic Indications[25]	Potential Side Effects[25]

Gentian Violet $C_{25}H_{30}ClN_3$		1. Antibacterial
		   Mostly gram positive
		   MRSA
		2. Antifungal
		   Candida
		3. Antihelminthic
		4. Antitrypanosomal
		   Transmission prevention
		5. Histologic stain
			1. Impetigo
			2. Infectious erosion
			3. Umbilical infection
			4. Infected ulcer
			5. Decubitus ulcer
			6. Angular cheilitis
			7. Paronychia
			8. MRSA nasal carriage
			9. Thrush
			   Especially in patients with human
			   immunodeficiency virus infection
				1. Contact dermatitis
				2. Mucosal irritation
				   Avoid eye or internal ear contact
				3. Necrotic skin reactions
				4. Leukopenia
				   When given intravenously
				5. Stains clothing, bedding

Brilliant Green $C_{27}H_{33}N_2 \cdot HO_4S$		1. Antiseptic 2. Antifungal Mycotic lung infections 3. Histologic stain	1. Paronychia 2. Infected wounds, burns	1. Contact dermatitis 2. Necrotic skin reactions 3. Stains clothing, bedding

Malachite Green
$C_{23}H_{25}ClN_2$

1. Antiseptic
   Mostly gram positive
2. Antifungal

1. Superficial pyodermas

1. Contact dermatitis
2. Stains clothing, bedding

Fuchsin
$C_{20}H_{20}N_3 \cdot HCl$

1. Antiseptics
   Gram positive
2. Antifungal
   Magenta paint,
   Castellani paint
3. Astringent
4. Histologic stain

1. Pyodermas
2. Dermatophytosis
3. Dermatitis
4. Intertrigo
5. Eczema
6. Burns

1. Contact dermatitis
2. Stains clothing, bedding

fallen out of favor in recent decades due in part to its cosmetic appearance as well as the concurrent increase of antibiotic use; it is of no coincidence that the last major human intervention trial with GV was in 1950, approximately 5 years after the development of mass production techniques for penicillin. Nevertheless, the utility of GV in a variety of infectious settings is well known to generations of physicians and mothers.

More pressingly, GV is active against MRSA in vitro[11]; its clinical utility was first demonstrated in a series of 14 patients with decubitus ulcers. Saji and colleagues[12] applied a 0.1% ointment of GV to the affected areas after patients had bathed in 0.1% solutions of GV. The average time to eradication of MRSA was 10.8 days ($\pm$2.7), while no patients experienced any appreciable side effects. Recently, Okano and colleagues[13] demonstrated the efficacy of GV in a broad range of MRSA SSTI and clearance of nasal carriage. In the 8 cases of impetigo, the mean time to eradication was 6.8 days ($\pm$3.7, range 4–15) and the in vitro minimum inhibitory concentration) of GV was 0.0225 μg/mL. The agent was well tolerated in all 37 patients, with no significant side effects being reported.

In the setting of secondary skin infections, the authors' group has recently reported a case in a patient with impetiginized eczema unresponsive to conventional therapy who showed dramatic clinical and symptomatic improvement with a combination of oral doxycycline and daily applications of GV.[14] This result builds on the work of Brockow and colleagues[15] who previously demonstrated the efficacy of GV alone in clearing *S aureus* from colonized lesions of atopic eczema. A 0.3% solution of GV was applied twice daily to lesional and nonlesional skin for 4 days and, compared with topical steroids and tar preparations, was the only agent to immediately reduce bacterial density at both sites ($P<.001$). GV not only helped clearing bacterial presence but also significantly reduced eczema severity.

Several hypotheses have been proposed to explain the bacteriostatic and bacteriocidal properties of GV, but the exact mechanisms remain unknown.[16] Nonetheless, given its low cost (US $0.08 per mL of a 2% solution),[17] ease of application, and clinical efficacy, GV must be considered as a legitimate treatment option in SSTI, particularly in the face of continued and emerging bacterial resistance.

REDUCING VASCULAR LEAK

The ability of the immune system to respond to bacterial insult is intimately tied to the ability of both serous and cellular elements to translocate across the vascular wall. The phenomenon of vascular leak is clinically evident in any erythematous or edematous lesion, including pyodermas. There are several signaling molecules responsible for this phenomenon, but the one of particular interest is angiopoietin-2 (ang-2), which is a 66-kDa protein stored in the Weibel-Palade bodies (WPB) of endothelial cells. On binding with the Tie2 receptor (a tyrosine kinase), ang-2 mediates endothelial cell activation and angiogenesis in addition to vascular permeability.[18] Several factors cause the release of ang-2 from the WPB, including thrombin, histamine, epinephrine, vascular endothelial growth factor, and hypoxia, elements that abound in injured or infected sites.[19]

Whereas vascular leak is integral to the immune response, it limits the accumulation of antibiotics at the sites of infection. Because serous fluid continues to accumulate in the so-called third space, antibiotics are delivered into edematous tissue at concentrations that are increasingly less than the required levels for activity. This effect is particularly evident in extreme situations such as fulminate sepsis in which diminished peripheral vascular resistance and vascular leak lead to tremendous third spacing of fluid—antibiotics are rendered less effective simply because they cannot reach appropriate drug levels. Serum levels of ang-2 have been shown to increase in overwhelming sepsis in a manner that correlates directly with the degree of sepsis and inversely with nitric oxide—dependent microvascular reactivity.[20] Particular to SSTI, the authors' group has recently demonstrated the elaboration of ang-2 in the wall of a staphylococcal abscess.[21] While the degree of impaired antibiotic delivery has yet to be determined in the setting of an abscess or other pyodermas, similar mechanisms in other disease states and the presence of ang-2 in SSTI lesions suggest a role.

Direct inhibitors of ang-2 are yet to be developed, but nitric oxide and hydrogen peroxide are 2 naturally occurring compounds that block the release of ang-2 from endothelial WPB.[22] On the synthetic front, the authors' group has demonstrated the utility of triphenylmethane dyes in reducing intratumor levels of ang-2 expression in a murine model. After establishment of a bEnd.3-derived hemangioma, mice were exposed to solutions of either GV or brilliant green (BG) via intralesional injections at 2 separate times over the course of 20 days. No significant side effects were noted throughout the trial, and, after killing, tumors in the GV and BG treatment groups were found to be 95.7% and 92.6% smaller (respectively) than the control vehicle group. In vivo exposure of bEnd.3 cells to GV and BG resulted in reductions of ang-2 expression to 30% and undetectable levels, respectively.[23] Clinically, while systematic trials are yet to be done, the authors have demonstrated the effectiveness of topically applied eosin (another triphenylmethane dye) in combination with pulsed dye laser, hydrocolloid dressings, or antibiotics in the treatment of 18 pediatric cases of ulcerated infantile hemangioma. Complete ulcer healing occurred in 16 patients after 4 weeks of therapy. In vitro, the treatment of bEnd.3 hemangioma cells with eosin resulted in significant decreases in levels of ang-2 expression.[24] Applying these data to pyodermas, administration of GV or other similar triphenylmethanes in combination with antibiotic therapy may act to reduce vascular leak and allow for improved antibiotic delivery.

RELATED COMPOUNDS

Other triphenylmethanes, in addition to GV, have had historical medical uses, mainly as histologic stains and antibacterial and antifungal agents; these agents included BG, malachite green, and fuchsin.[8,25] Their therapeutic applications are known mainly through case reports, with a notable paucity of systematic clinical trials when compared with GV. See **Table 1** for a summary of the known uses.

REFERENCES

1. Graham PL 3rd, Lin SX, Larson EL. A U.S. population-based survey of Staphylococcus aureus colonization. Ann Intern Med 2006;144(5):318–25.
2. Odell CA. Community-associated methicillin-resistant Staphylococcus aureus (CA-MRSA) skin infections. Curr Opin Pediatr 2010;22(3):273–7.
3. Cooke FJ, Brown NM. Community-associated methicillin-resistant Staphylococcus aureus infections. Br Med Bull 2010;94:215–27.
4. Sánchez García M, De la Torre MA, Morales G, et al. Clinical outbreak of linezolid-resistant Staphylococcus aureus in an intensive care unit. JAMA 2010;303(22):2260–4.
5. Shrand H. Thrush in the newborn. Br Med J 1961;2:1530–3.
6. Harvey SC. Antiseptics and disinfectants; fungicides; ectoparasiticides. In: Goodman LS, Gilman A, editors. The pharmacological basis of therapeutics. New York: Macmillan; 1975. p. 987–1017.
7. Wald ER, Snyder MJ, Gutberlet RL. Group B beta-hemolytic streptococcal colonization: acquisition, persistence, and effect of umbilical cord treatment with triple dye. Am J Dis Child 1977;131:178–80.
8. Bakker P, van Doorne H, Gooskens V, et al. Activity of gentian violet and brilliant green against some microorganisms associated with skin infections. Int J Dermatol 1992;31:210–3.
9. Churchman JW. The selective bactericidal action of gentian violet. J Exp Med 1912;16:221–47.
10. Hinton D. Results of the intravenous use of gentian violet in cases of extreme septicemia. Ann Surg 1925;81(3):687–92.
11. Saji M. [Effect of gentiana violet against methicillin-resistant Staphylococcus aureus (MRSA)]. Kansen-shogaku Zasshi 1994;66:914–22 [in Japanese].
12. Saji M, Taguchi S, Uchiyama K, et al. Efficacy of gentian violet in the eradication of methicillin-resistant Staphylococcus aureus from skin lesions. J Hosp Infect 1995;31:225–8.
13. Okano M, Noguchi S, Tabata K, et al. Topical gentian violet for cutaneous infection and nasal carriage with MRSA. Int J Dermatol 2000;39(12):942–4.
14. Arbiser JL, MacKelfresh J, Stoff B. A nonsteroidal alternative to impetiginized eczema in the emergency room. J Amer Acad Dermatol 2010;63(3):537–9.
15. Brockow K, Grabenhorst P, Abeck D, et al. Effect of gentian violet, corticosteroid and tar preparations in Staphylococcus-aureus-colonized atopic eczema. Dermatology 1999;199(3):231–6.
16. Docampo R, Moreno SNJ. The metabolism and mode of action of gentian violet. Drug Metab Rev 1990;22:161–6.
17. Available at: http://www.amazon.com/GENTIAN-VIOLET-SOL-2-HUM/dp/B000GCQ05G. Accessed July 23, 2010.
18. Fiedler U, Augustin HG. Angiopoietins: a link between angiogenesis and inflammation. Trends Immunol 2006;27:552–8.
19. Lowenstein CJ, Morrell CN, Yamakuchi M. Regulation of Weibel-Palade body exocytosis. Trends Cardiovasc Med 2005;15:302–8.
20. Davis JS, Yeo TW, Piera KA, et al. Angiopoietin-2 is increased in sepsis and inversely associated with nitric oxide-dependent microvascular reactivity. Crit Care 2010;14(3):R89.
21. Arbiser JL. High level expression of angiopoietin-2 in human abscesses. J Amer Acad Dermatol, in press.
22. Matsushita K, Morrell CN, Cambien B, et al. Nitric oxide regulates exocytosis by S-nitrosylation of N-ethylmaleimide-sensitive factor. Cell 2003;115:139–50.
23. Perry BN, Govindarajan B, Bhandarkar SS, et al. Pharmacologic blockade of angiopoietin-2 is efficacious against model hemangiomas in mice. J Invest Dermatol 2006;126(10):2316–22.
24. Lapidoth M, Ben-Amitai D, Bhandarkar S, et al. Efficacy of topical application of eosin for ulcerated hemangiomas. J Am Acad Dermatol 2009;60(2):350–1.
25. Balabanova M, Popova L, Tchipeva R. Dyes in dermatology. Clin Dermatol 2003;21(1):2–6.

Cutaneous Leishmaniasis in Mali

Carlos Paz, MD, PhD[a],*, Seydou Doumbia, MD, PhD[b],
Somita Keita, MD[c], Aisha Sethi, MD[a]

KEYWORDS

• *Leishmania major* • Cutaneous leishmaniasis • Mali

Leishmaniasis is a disease caused by obligate intracellular protozoan parasites belonging to the genus *Leishmania,* and it is transmitted by the bite of female phlebotomine sand flies. More than 20 *Leishmania* parasite species cause human disease. Depending on the causative agent, disease manifests as visceral, cutaneous, or mucocutaneous forms. In the most severe form of the disease, visceral leishmaniasis, the parasite migrates to internal organs such as the liver and spleen and can be fatal if left untreated. Mucocutaneous leishmaniasis results in disfiguring lesions of the nose, mouth, and throat mucous membranes. Cutaneous leishmaniasis, the most common form of the disease, is characterized by painless skin ulcerations usually on exposed areas such as the face and extremities.[1] The lesions of cutaneous leishmaniasis develop at site of inoculation after an incubation period of weeks to months. Initially, the lesions are painless erythematous papules that become darker and develop a crust in the center over the course of several weeks. Eventually, the center of the lesion ulcerates, and the edges become raised. In 3 to 6 months, the lesions heal, leaving behind depigmented retracted scars (**Fig. 1**).[1]

Cutaneous leishmaniasis can be found in at least 88 countries, and it affects as many as 12 million people worldwide, with 1.5 to 2 million new cases every year.[2] The disease is found in tropical and subtropical countries, from the rainforests of Central and South America to the deserts of West Africa and the Middle East. Cutaneous leishmaniasis is divided into Old World (including southern Europe, the Middle East, parts of southwest Asia and Africa) and New World (from the southern United States through Latin America to South America) forms based on geographic setting of the infection. Both Old World leishmaniasis and New World cutaneous leishmaniasis are caused by distinct vectors and sets of parasites. For example, New World infection is transmitted by the sand flies belonging to the genus *Lutzomyia,* whereas Old World disease is transmitted by sand flies belonging to the genus *Phlebotomus.*[1] *Leishmania mexicana, L brazilensis,* and *L amazonensis* parasite species cause New World cutaneous leishmaniasis, and *L major, L tropica, L aethiopica,* and *L infantum* parasite species cause Old World cutaneous leishmaniasis.[1]

CUTANEOUS LEISHMANIASIS IN MALI
Mali

Mali is a land-locked country in West Africa, surrounded by seven countries including Algeria, Burkina Fasso, Guinea, Ivory Coast, Mauritania, Niger, and Senegal. Mali extends southwest from the arid southern Sahara through the semiarid Sahel to the Sudanian savannah. Mali has a diverse population of over 12 million people, composed of at least six different ethnic groups.[3] Approximately three quarters of its population live in rural areas, and roughly 10% are nomadic. Historically, Mali was at the center of the trans-Saharan gold and salt trade connecting North Africa to sub-Saharan Africa. This historical connection almost certainly accounts for the fact that approximately 90% of Malians are Muslim today.[3] Mali was colonized by the French between 1892 and 1960. Despite nearly

[a] Section of Dermatology, University of Chicago, 5841 South Maryland Avenue, MC 5067, Chicago, IL 60637, USA
[b] Malaria Research Training Center, University of Bamako, Bamako, Mali
[c] Centre National d'Appui a la lutte contre la Maladie (CNAM), Bamako, Mali
* Corresponding author.
E-mail address: Carlos.Paz@uchospitals.edu

Dermatol Clin 29 (2011) 75–78
doi:10.1016/j.det.2010.08.013

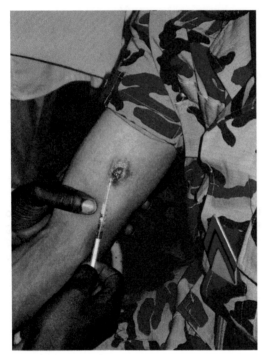

Fig. 1. A polymerase chain reaction-confirmed case of cutaneous leishmaniasis in Mali.

a half century as an independent state, the official language is still French, but the vast majority of Malians communicate in local African dialects, the most common being Bambara. Mali remains among the lowest ranking country in the world with regard to education and health indicators. The adult literacy rate ranges between 30% to 40%.[3] Roughly 40% of the population do not have access to safe drinking water.[3] The life expectancy is approximately 49 years, and the infant mortality rate is greater than 106 deaths per 1000 live births.[3] In general, access to professional health care is limited, and many Malians still treat ailments with traditional remedies. Limited health resources have made it difficult for scientists to obtain accurate data regarding the prevalence and incidence of diseases, especially those that are not life-threatening like cutaneous leishmaniasis.

Epidemiology

The first report of cutaneous leishmaniasis in Mali dates back to 1948 when Lefrou described two cases from Nioro, a town near the Mauritania border.[4] Ten years later, two foci of cutaneous leishmaniasis were identified in the western and central part of the country.[5] In the 1960s, nearly 600 cases of cutaneous leishmaniasis were reported in six different regions, expanding the total area containing the disease to most of the country.[6]

More recently, Keita and colleagues[7] reported on 251 cases of cutaneous leishmaniasis from throughout Mali. While the first reports of cutaneous leishmaniasis in Mali came from archives of medical records, the first objective data regarding the epidemiology of the disease were established between 1969 and 1970, when Imperato and colleagues[6,8–11] used the leishmanin skin test to show that the disease was present in most parts of the country, particularly in the Sahel. One study reported that the condition was slightly more common in males compared with females, 21.1% and 15.1% respectively, and that 18.1% of the subjects had contracted the disease at some point during their lives.[6] Moreover, of the subjects studied (mostly school-aged children), a higher percentage of older individuals were positive. A more recent study on the epidemiology of cutaneous leishmaniasis in two neighboring villages in central Mali confirmed Imperato's prevalence findings in one village (19.9% in Sougoula) but showed a twofold higher prevalence in the other village (45.4% in Kemena).[12] The same study also showed a difference in the incidence of Leishmania infection between Kemena and Sougula, approximately 18% and 6%, respectively. The prevalence and incidence findings of this study also illustrated an interesting phenomenon long known about cutaneous leishmaniasis; two foci as close as a few kilometers apart can have disparate prevalence and incidence statistics. Among other factors, the difference can likely be accounted for by the availability of infected reservoirs at each locus.

Leishmania Parasite

More than 20 Leishmania species cause human infection. L major, L tropica, L aethiopica, and L infantum parasite species cause Old World cutaneous leishmaniasis.[1] Of all the Old World Leishmania parasite species, only L major has been found in Mali. Before 2009, L major had been isolated from only two patients in Mali, one a tourist and the other a native of the country.[13,14] A more recent study identified four different L major strains in Mali.[15] While these reports established the presence of L major in Mali, they did not address whether L major is the only parasite species in the country, nor did they provide information on the geographic distribution of the parasite. Indeed, reports from countries adjacent to Mali have shown that parasite species other than L major can transmit cutaneous leishmaniasis.[16] To address these questions, scientists in Mali are amplifying Leishmania DNA from skin scrapings of approximately one hundred cutaneous leishmaniasis patients from different regions of the country. Their study is designed to distinguish between parasite species on the basis of the size of the resultant PCR product and by DNA sequencing. Based on published reports, *L major* may be the predominant, if not exclusive species responsible for cutaneous leishmaniasis in Mali.[13–15] However, given the diversity of geographic and eco-climatic zones, it is possible that other parasite species will be detected.[16]

Vector

For the most part, cutaneous leishmaniasis is a disease of animals but affects people when sand flies, the animal reservoir, and humans coexist. Female phlebotomine sand flies transmit cutaneous leishmaniasis to people. In West Africa, two main genera of sand flies exist, *Phlebotomus* and *Sergentomyia*.[17] Whereas *Phlebotomus* sand flies are known vectors of cutaneous leishmaniasis, *Sergentomyia* sand flies do not generally transmit the disease.[18] In a focus of infection in neighboring Senegal, *Phlebotomus duboscqi* was identified as the vector for cutaneous leishmaniasis.[19] Consistent with what is known about sand fly genera in West Africa, members of the *Phlebotomus* genera, including *P duboscqi*, have been found in Mali.[20,21] A study of possible vectors in Mali found *P duboscqi* throughout every region of the country,[21] while a more recent study recorded *P duboscqi* in Kemena, a village with active cases of cutaneous leishmaniasis.[12,20] While the presence of *P duboscqi* sand flies in Mali is well established, to date there have been no reports of *Leishmania*-infected sand flies collected in the country. Malian scientists are now actively involved in an effort to characterize the diversity of sand fly species in villages with active cases of the disease. Moreover, they have started to utilize molecular biology techniques, including PCR to detect infected sand flies. If the prevalence and incidence studies are correct,[12] it should not be long before they definitely identify the vector in Mali.

Reservoir

Throughout the world, nonhuman mammals, especially dogs and rodents, are reservoirs of cutaneous leishmaniasis. People, it turns out, are not good reservoirs.[18] In the early 1980s, rodent species *Mastomys erythroleucus, Tatera gambiana,* and *Arvicanthis niloticus* and a dog were identified as the bearers of *Leishmania* parasites in Senegal and Gambia.[22–26] While dogs are certainly commonplace in Mali, they are not as common as rodents. Indeed, a multitude of rodent species can be found in Mali,[27] including those known to be vectors of cutaneous leishmaniasis

in the neighboring country of Senegal. The reservoir of cutaneous leishmaniasis in Mali has (have) not been identified. Given the promiscuity of Leishmania parasites toward mammalian hosts, any number of the mammalian species in Mali could theoretically serve as the reservoir. Malian scientists have made limited, but unsuccessful, attempts at identifying Leishmania-infected rodents in villages with active cases of cutaneous leishmaniasis. Until an infected non-human mammal is identified, the reservoir in Mali will remain unknown.

SUMMARY

Information about cutaneous leishmaniasis in Mali is sparse. For nearly half a century, scientists have known that cutaneous leishmaniasis is prevalent in Mali, yet to this date there is little to no information regarding the vector, reservoir, and diversity of parasite species responsible for disease in that country. Studies have identified *L major* as the causative agent of at least some cases of cutaneous leishmaniasis in Mali. *P duboscqi*, a vector for cutaneous leishmaniasis in neighboring Senegal, has long been known to be present in Mali; however, infected sand flies have yet to be documented. Mali is rife with small mammals, many of which can be potential reservoirs, yet an infected reservoir has not been identified. Malian scientists, in collaboration with scientists in the United States, have initiated studies to address these questions.

REFERENCES

1. Herwaldt BL. Leishmaniasis. Lancet 1999;354: 1191–9.
2. Centers for Disease Control and Prevention. *Leishmania* infection fact sheet. Atlanta (GA); Centers for Disease Control and Prevention. Available at: http://www.cdc.gov/ncidod/dpd/parasites/leishmania/factsht_leishmania.htm. Accessed August 27, 2010.
3. Central Intelligence Agency (CIA). World factbook. Central Intelligence Agency. Available at: https://www.cia.gov/library/publications/the-world-factbook/geos/ml.html. Accessed August 27, 2010.
4. Lefrou G. La Leishmaniose cutanee au Soudan francais. Frequence de la forme seche papulo-tuberculeuse. Bull Soc Path Exot 1948;41:622–7.
5. Sankale M, Le Viguelloux J, Rivoalen A, et al. Bull Soc Pathol Exot Filiales 1958;51:203–9.
6. Imperato PJ, Diakite S. Leishmaniasis in the republic of Mali. Trans R Soc Trop Med Hyg 1969; 63:236–41.
7. Keita S, Faye O, Ndiaye Ht, et al. Epidemiologie et polymorphisme clinique de la leishmaniose cutanee

observe au CNAM (ex-Institut Marchoux) Bamako (Mali). Mali Medical 2003;XVIII:29–31.

8. Imperato PJ, Bradrick M. Leishmanin skin sensitivity in Timbuctoo. J Trop Med Hyg 1969;72:216–8.

9. Imperato PJ, Coulibaly B, Togola T. Leishmanin skin sensitivity in northwestern Mali. Acta Trop 1970;27:260–5.

10. Imperato PJ, Sow O, Fofana B. Positive leishmanin skin sensitivity in the absence of clinical leishmaniasis. J Trop Med Hyg 1973;76:132–4.

11. Imperato PJ, Fofana B, Sow O, et al. Leishmanin skin sensitivity in the inland delta of the Niger. Trop Geogr Med 1974;26:303–6.

12. Oliveira F, Doumbia S, Anderson JM, et al. Discrepant prevalence and incidence of leishmania infection between two neighboring villages in Central Mali based on Leishmanin skin test surveys. PLoS Negl Trop Dis 2009;3:e565.

13. Garin JP, Peyramond D, Piens MA, et al. Presence of Leishmania major Yakimoff and Schokhor, 1914 in Mali. Enzymatic identification of a strain of human origin. Ann Parasitol Hum Comp 1985;60:93–4.

14. Izri MA, Doumbo O, Belazzoug S, et al. Presence of Leishmania major MON-26 in Mali. Ann Parasitol Hum Comp 1989;64:510–1.

15. Pratlong F, Dereure J, Ravel C, et al. Geographical distribution and epidemiological features of old world cutaneous leishmaniasis foci, based on the isoenzyme analysis of 1048 strains. Trop Med Int Health 2009;14:1071–85.

16. Milhoubi I, Picot S, Hafirassou N, et al. Cutaneous leishmaniasis caused by Leishmania tropica in Algeria. Trans R Soc Trop Med Hyg 2008;102:1157–9.

17. Boakye D, Wilson M, Kweku M. A review of leishmaniasis in West Africa. Ghana Med J 2005;39:94–7.

18. Lawyer PG, Ngumbi PM, Anjili CO, et al. Development of Leishmania major in Phlebotomus duboscqi and Sergentomyia schwetzi (Diptera: Psychodidae). Am J Trop Med Hyg 1990;43(1):31–43.

19. Dedet JP, Saf Janova VM, Desjeux P, et al. Ecology of a reservoir of cutaneous lieshmaniasis in the region of Thies (Senegal, West Africa). Characterization and types of isolates Leishmania strains. Bull Soc Pathol Exot Filiales 1982;75:155–68.

20. Kato H, Anderson JM, Kamhawi S, et al. High degree of conservancy among secreted salivary gland proteins from two geographically distant Phlebotomus duboscqi sandflies populations (Mali and Kenya). BMC Genomics 2006;4;7:226.

21. Lariviere M, Abonnenc E, Kramer R. [Chronicle of cutaneous leishmaniasis in West Africa. The problem of the vector]. Bulletin de la Societe de pathologie exotique et de ses filiales 1961;54:1031–46 [in French].

22. Bjorvatn B, Neva FA. A model in mice for experimental leishmaniasis with a West African strain of Leishmania tropica. Am J Trop Med Hyg 1979;28:472–9.

23. Blanchot M, Lusina D, Beunier E. Interepidemic surveillance of a cutaneous leishmaniasis focus in Senegal. Med Trop 1984;44:35–40.

24. Dedet JP, Hubert B, Desjeux F, et al. Ecology of a cutaneous leishmaniasis focus in the Thies region (Senegal, West Africa). Spontaneous infection and disease reservoir role of various wild rodent species. Bull Soc Pathol Exot Filiales 1981;74:71–7.

25. Dedet JP, Desjeux P, Derouin F. Ecology of a cutaneous leishmaniasis focus in the Thies region (Senegal, West Africa). Spontaneous infestation and biology of Phlebotomus duboscqi Neveu-Lemaire 1906. Bull Soc Pathol Exot Filiales 1982;75:588–98.

26. Desjeux P, Bryan JH, Martin-Saxton P. Leishmaniasis in the Gambia. 2. A study of possible vectors and animal reservoirs, with the first report of a case of canine leishmaniasis in the Gambia. Trans R Soc Trop Med Hyg 1983;77:143–8.

27. The IUCN Red List of Threatened Species: Mammals of Mali. IUCN; 2010. Available at: www.iucnredlist.org. Accessed August 27, 2010.

Albinism in Africa: Stigma, Slaughter and Awareness Campaigns

Andres E. Cruz-Inigo, MD[a], Barry Ladizinski, MD[b], Aisha Sethi, MD[c],*

KEYWORDS

- Albinism • Sub-Saharan Africa • Albino murders
- Albino slaughters • Albinism myths
- Albinism awareness campaigns

Originating from the word "albus," meaning white in Latin, albinism is a genetic disorder resulting in a decrease or absence of pigmentation in the hair, eyes, and skin.[1,2] The prevalence of oculocutaneous albinism (OCA) is about 1:37,000 in the United States[3] and 1:20,000 in most populations in the world.[4] The prevalence in regions of sub-Saharan Africa is estimated to be much greater than these figures; for example, it is estimated at about 1:4000 in Zimbabwe[3] and in Tanzania it is 1:1429.[5] Albinism most commonly arises from mutations in genes encoding for proteins involved in the synthesis or transport of melanin by melanocytes. As well as giving skin its color, melanin protects the skin from the deleterious effects of the sun's ultraviolet radiation (UVR) and, although present, melanocytes in OCA are dysfunctional, predisposing individuals to cutaneous and ocular pathologic conditions. This is particularly problematic for albinos living in South Africa who suffer both emotionally and physically from dermatologic malignancies and, more recently, must cope with being hunted for their body parts as well. Thus, it is imperative to inform the medical community and the general national and international public about the tragedies faced by albinos to protect them from skin cancer and ritualistic murders by individuals seeking wealth through clandestine markets perpetuating witchcraft.[6]

DEMYSTIFYING ALBINISM MYTHS AND MISCONCEPTIONS

Throughout Africa, an indeterminate number of individuals with albinism, especially children, have been the victims of brutal attacks and murder in the name of witchcraft, superstition, and wealth (**Box 1**). Most recently, the atrocities committed against albinos has received widespread attention because of various crimes reported, such as infanticide, kidnapping, amputations, and decapitations, committed for purposes of supplying highly valued body parts used for amulets, which are then sold in underground witchcraft markets. For example, up to $75,000 may be offered for a set of arms, legs, ears, and genitals from an individual with albinism.[6] Thus, albinos must live in a constant state of guilt and angst, often forced to flee their homes and live in solitude to avoid the albino hunters. The main driving forces underlying these profiling crimes are ignorance, myth, and superstition, such as the belief that individuals

Funding sources: none.

Disclosures: the authors have nothing to disclose.

[a] Scripps Mercy Hospital, 4280 Arguello Street, San Diego, CA 92103, USA

[b] Department of Internal Medicine, Yale University School of Medicine, 333 Cedar Street, 1074 LMP, PO Box 208030, New Haven, CT 06520-8030, USA

[c] Section of Dermatology, University of Chicago, 5841 South Maryland Avenue MC 5067, Chicago, IL 60637, USA

* Corresponding author.

E-mail address: asethi@medicine.bsd.uchicago.edu

Dermatol Clin 29 (2011) 79–87

doi:10.1016/j.det.2010.08.015

0733-8635/11/$ — see front matter © 2011 Published by Elsevier Inc.

Box 1
Common myths and misconceptions regarding albinism

Weaving albino hair into a net improves the chances of catching fish

Albino body parts worn as amulets bring good luck, fortune, and health

Albino body parts are a necessary ingredient for witchdoctor potions

Albinos have magical superpowers and can cure diseases

Intercourse with an albino lady will cure human immunodeficiency virus (HIV) infection

Spitting on an albino prevents the condition in one's family

Mother of albino child was laughed at by an albino during pregnancy

Albinism is caused by a missing top layer of skin

Albinos and their mothers are possessed by evil spirits

The devil stole the original child and replaced it with an albino

Albinism is very contagious and spread through touching

Albinos are housed by ghosts of European colonists

Albinos have low brain capacity and cannot function at the same level as others

Mother of albino was impregnated by a white man

with albinism possess superpowers or that their body parts bestow fortune and health.[7] Thus, the stigma and atrocities affecting the albino population may be attributed to lack of familiarity and education about albinism coupled with ignorance. Compared with albinos in developed countries, many albinos in sub-Saharan Africa suffer from a lack of access to health care and awareness within their communities of their condition. This may manifest itself in a higher and earlier incidence of skin cancer, mortality, and stigmatization.

Based primarily on its major pattern of autosomal recessive inheritance, the prevalence, morbidity, and mortality of albinism could be diminished with the education of school-aged children, particularly emphasizing the consequences of marrying relatives. Although many of the genetic causes and inheritance patterns of albinism have been established, many communities are uninformed and unaware of the implications of such consanguineous matrimonial arrangements.[3]

Thus, the high incidence of OCA in certain regions of sub-Saharan Africa might be due to encouragement of consanguineous alliances.[3] For instance, some of the coastal communities in Tanzania "are matrilineal. Children of a maternal uncle belong to the clan of the wife of that uncle and therefore to a different clan from the children of his sisters and brothers. First cousins may therefore marry, enhancing the chances of albino offspring. Compounding this is the influence on coastal people of the Arab tradition of marrying among relatives, so that family property remains within the clan."[8]

These practices inevitably increase the incidence of albinism amongst children of related parents. Nevertheless, the traditional consanguineous marriage arrangements are not the only reason for the high prevalence of albinism in certain regions, as "communities may have fewer cases to show because many areas still practice infanticide. Traditional midwives may sometimes kill off albino children and the case is then presented as a stillbirth."[8] Such evidence further highlights the prevalence of severe stigmas and misconceptions associated with albinism and the need for improved awareness.

Tanzanians as well as other sub-Saharan Africans believe in numerous myths and superstitions regarding the etiology of albinism, unaware of its genetic cause, and further contributing to its high incidence. For example, Lund surveyed 138 schoolchildren (average age 14.4 years old) with albinism in Zimbabwe about the cause of OCA, and found that 70 (50.7%) had no knowledge of why they lacked skin coloration and were different from their classmates, 15 (10.9%) favored a biologic reason, 19 (13.8%) believed God was responsible, and 13 (9.4%) stated other incorrect causes, such as witchery, punishment for a family member mocking an albino and "top layer of skin missing."[3] Other misconceptions regarding the cause of albinism include the belief that the mother was impregnated by a white man or that the devil replaced the African child with an albino.[2]

Furthermore, although more than 50% of albinos in Tanzania have an albino relative, most do not recognize its genetic cause.[2] In a study assessing albino attitudes and beliefs, McBride and Leppard[9] demonstrated that although 59 participants with OCA had an albino relative, only 13 believed that the condition was inherited. In some regions, the misconceptions about the cause of albinism might extend into the health care field to include physicians and nurses, who may be under the impression that albinism is contagious and therefore might avoid physical and social contact with those affected.[3]

In addition to the distinct physical features of albinism, the social structure and superstitious belief system provides the grounds for further prejudice and social rejection. In Zimbabwe, albinos are called "sope," which suggests that they are inhabited by evil spirits; in Tanzania, they are also ridiculed and called "nguruwe," which means pig; "zeru," which means ghost; or "mzungu," which means white person.[2,10] Beginning in childhood, their marked and dissimilar exterior appearance compared with "normally pigmented family members and the rest of the black community, results in problems of acceptance and social integration for those affected."[3,11–15]

Lund[16] reported that albino students in a school in Zimbabwe were not only called names and ridiculed, but were also beaten and avoided by peers who would not eat or play with them. Some participants in this study reported that they were mocked and avoided by family members, who would not share food or clothes with their albino relatives. Many albino children were not allowed to visit their parents' workplaces and were sometimes placed in the sun to become accustomed to UVR.[6] Thus, it is not surprising, that one 15-year-old albino confessed, "I cannot see the blackboard clearly. I cannot work in the open doing manual work. I don't like walking long distances to interschool sports. I am always being humiliated by others calling me names."[16] Although some albinos may benefit from a good family support system, once they leave home many encounter rejection by employers[16] in what some have described as "apartheid in reverse."[8] The superstitions surrounding albinism may also place mothers of albinos in a vulnerable position, subject to stigmatization and harassment, and resulting in severe psychosocial distress.[1]

As the general medical term implies, OCA also affects the eyes; some studies have indicated that up to 100% of albinos have some form of visual impairment.[17,18] Ocular disorders associated with OCA include hypopigmentation of the iris and retina, hypoplastic fovea, hyperopia, strabismus, photophobia, loss of stereoscopic perception, and nystagmus.[2] Such visual handicaps hinder some of the major components of learning, such as reading and seeing the blackboard. These obstacles place albino students at a disadvantage, as many cannot afford ophthalmic care or appropriate visual aids. Visual impairments, poverty, lack of access to health care, and that lack of educational provisions inevitably result in poor educational outcomes and continued frustration. Consequently, this fosters a cycle that prevents albinos from succeeding and condemns them to manual outdoor labor,

such as that in sisal plantations, further increasing the risk for skin damage.

Because of a lack of melanin, which serves as the skin's own sunscreen against UVR, albinos are predisposed to various types of solar skin damage, such as actinic cheilitis, actinic keratoses, and various skin cancers.[2] The likelihood of damage increases in tropical climate regions, as the amount of clothing worn is typically minimal while the daily exposure to UVR is maximal. Studies have shown that the risk for dermatologic malignancy in sun-exposed areas (such as the face, ears, neck, and shoulders) is enhanced in individuals with OCA, who may present with solar keratoses as early as 8 years of age.[1,2,17]

A study amongst individuals with OCA in Tanzania revealed that 100% exhibited skin damage by the first year of life and advanced symptomatic cancers were observed in 50% of those between 20 and 30 years of age, with 1 case of skin cancer in a 9-year-old child.[19] In a Nigerian study, no albinos older than 20 years of age were free of subclinical malignant skin damage and in the 1980s, less than 10% of albinos living around Dar es Salaam survived beyond 30 years of age. Within Tanzania, less than 2% of albino children were expected to reach 40 years of age.[6,19] A more recent study conducted in northern Tanzania reported that although albinos previously died between 20 and 30 years of age, today they live considerably longer because of preventive sun protection.[2] Nevertheless, in regions afflicted by poverty, sunscreens are unaffordable and only available to a limited portion of the population; thus, strategies should focus on sun avoidance and other means of protection early in childhood.[15,16]

During the 1980s in Dar es Salaam, individuals suffering from albinism had about 4 years between the presentation of irreversible skin pathology and metastatic disease, mainly caused by squamous cell carcinoma (SCC) in the head and neck region.[19] Lack of access to medical care or neglect might be one of the reasons why skin cancer has a deadlier course in the albino population near the Equator than in other developed countries.[19] Mortality from SCC is low amongst fair-skinned individuals in developed, equatorial nations with high levels of UVR, but amongst albinos in Nigeria and Tanzania, it is very high.

The low life expectancy in the albino population is clearly multifactorial. Those suffering from albinism are often unable to succeed in school. One study reported that only 12 of 350 adults with OCA worked indoors, suggesting that outdoor occupations are contributing to the lower life expectancy for albinos.[19] As previously mentioned, albinos are often discriminated against and the system in place does not have the educational provisions to address their poor eyesight and allow them to succeed and compete with the nonalbino population. For example, in his editorial article, "White skin, black souls", Kuster[10] indicates that in Malawi, "it is a common belief that albinos have low brain capacity and are unable to function at the same level as 'normal people'." Kuster[10] further notes than an educated albino woman never held a job in Zimbabwe because "employers always said, more or less, during the interview that an albino secretary would hurt the company's reputation" because of the fear that albinism is contagious.

The first step in assisting individuals with albinism in sub-Saharan Africa would be to educate the population as a whole about the cause of albinism and decrease prevalence by increasing awareness of the implications of consanguineous relationships (**Box 2**). Poverty and illiteracy in some parts of Africa may result in a lack of understanding among individuals that marriage between cousins can increase the chances of acquiring certain genetic disorders.[2] Raising awareness through radio broadcasts and schools' curricula might be helpful in promoting integration, albeit challenging, given that albinism is steeped in superstition and misconceptions that lead to fear and misunderstanding.[3] Albinos and parents of albino children must understand the causes of albinism, its many medical and psychosocial implications, and how to appropriately protect themselves from UVR. In particular, the benefits of sun protection and the consequences of solar

injury should be stressed, as studies have shown that many albinos are not familiar with this information. For example, in a study by McBride and Leppard,[9] 10% of albinos surveyed stated that they only applied sunscreen at night and some did not wear sun-protective clothing, such as wide-brimmed hats, because of fashion and cultural concerns. It is also imperative that mothers of newborns with albinism fully understand the cause before returning home from the hospital, as members of the family and community may assume that the infant is of uncertain ancestry, resulting in condemnation of the mother and rejection of the child.[14] Teachers must be informed that children with albinism are as capable as other students, but have difficulties with vision and reading, thus requiring enlarged text textbooks and seating closer to the blackboard.[2]

In the clinical setting, individuals with albinism should be provided with dermatologic examinations, guidelines on how to shield themselves from the sun, and sun protection products such as sunscreen, sunglasses, opaque clothing that covers most of the skin, scarves, high socks, and wide-brimmed hats. Given that most albinos are unemployed, they cannot afford sun-protective gear, which is expensive in Africa, thus it should be encouraged that society establish measures to support albinos and their families. Governmental endeavors may include assistance with indoor job placement, supplying adequate amounts of sun-protective products and funding for organizations involved in albinism awareness and support. Most of the educational provisions necessary for students with albinism are not being met, and in Tanzania, unlike Zimbabwe,[20] there are no provisions for children with visual problems or handicaps.[9] In the current circumstances, little can be accomplished without the government's support and international assistance. An unsupportive social environment hinders the progress of individuals with albinism, stagnating their intellectual and physical potential, despite their desire to progress.[21]

AWARENESS CAMPAIGNS

Recently, various organizations dedicated to increasing albinism awareness and assisting albinos in attaining proper medical care and appropriate sun protection have been established throughout the world (**Table 1**). For example, the Regional Dermatologic Training Center (RDTC) at the Kilimanjaro Christian Medical Center (KCMC) in Moshi, Tanzania, has created an albino assistance program and mobile skin care clinic.[9,22] The primary mission of the RDTC has been to

---

Box 2
Albino needs for improved survival

Sun protection education

Sun protection products

Eye care and corrective lenses

Wide-brimmed hats, sunglasses, scarves

Educational provisions

Magnifying glasses, braille machines

Opaque clothing and high socks

Regular full body skin checks

Indoor job placement assistance

Genetic transmission education

Enhanced protection from criminals

Swift justice for captured albino hunters

Awareness campaigns to debunk myths

Table 1
Albinism assistance and awareness organizations

Albinism Organizations	Contact Information
National Organization for Albinism and Hypopigmentation (NOAH)	http://www.albinism.org
Ghana Association of Persons Living with Albinism (GAPA)	http://www.gapagh.org/stigmatization.html
Tanzania Albino Center (TAC)	http://www.tanzaniaalbino.org/
Stichting Afrikaanse Albino (SAA)	http://www.afrikaansealbinos.nl
Assisting Children in Need (ACN)	http://www.assistingchildreninneed.com
Regional Dermatologic Training Center (RDTC)	http://gc21.inwent.org/ibt/site/rdtc/ibt/main.html
Albino Association of Malawi (TAAM)	http://www.fedoma.net/members/taam.php
Albinism Fellowship United Kingdom	http://www.albinism.org.uk/
Asante Mariamu	http://www.asante-mariamu.org
Tanzania Vision Support	http://www.thefoundation-tz.org
Positive Exposure	http://www.positiveexposure.org
Albinism Trust New Zealand	http://www.albinism.org.nz/home.html
Cordaid	http://www.cordaid.nl/
Under the Same Sun	http://www.underthesamesun.com/home.php
Albinism Fellowship of Australia	http://www.albinismaustralia.org/
ALBA (Asociación de Ayuda a Personas con Albinismo)	http://www.albinismo.es/
WHO Intersun Program	http://www.who.int/uv.
BaiChina (Kids from China with Albinism)	http://groups.yahoo.com/group/baichina/
Chicago Connection for Minorities with Albinism (CCM)	http://groups.yahoo.com/group/NOAH_CCMA/
Norwegian Association for Albinism (NFFA)	http://www.albinisme.no/
The Hermansky-Pudlak Syndrome (HPS) Network	http://www.hpsnetwork.org/

significantly improve the living conditions of albinos living in Tanzania. A physician and nurse in a 4-wheel drive vehicle regularly visit 10 villages within a100-km^2 area in Arusha and Kilimanjaro. During these visits, skin checks are performed and sun protection information and supplies are provided.[22]

Dr Aisha Sethi, an assistant professor of dermatology in the Pritzker School of Medicine, has dedicated her time to educating Malawians about albinism; she is specifically interested in eliminating the various superstitions surrounding OCA (**Fig. 1**).[23] In 2007, Sethi established the first albinism clinic in Malawi's capital, Lilongwe, and for the past 3 years has organized an annual Albino Awareness Day in Malawi, aimed at skin cancer screening, public education, and denouncing stigmas (**Fig. 2**). Dorothy Shope, an education coordinator in the University of Chicago Medical Center's dermatology section, recently recommended that the team provide albinos with magnifying glasses, a simple

and inexpensive solution for children without access to eye care or corrective lenses.[23]

Established in 2003, the Tanzania Albino Center (TAC) is an organization in Arusha, Tanzania; its

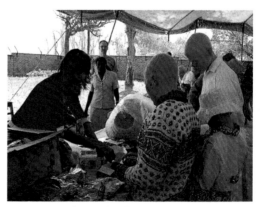

Fig. 1. Dr Aisha Sethi distributing sun protection products to children with albinism.

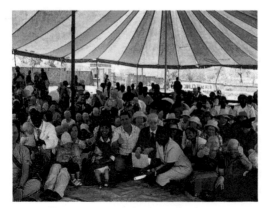

Fig. 2. Albino awareness day in Malawi.

aim is to improve the lives of albinos with educational and medical assistance so that they may live safe, accepted, and prosperous lives in the society of their choice.[24] In partnership with the Hands of Africa Foundation and the Dutch organization, Stichting Afrikaanse Albinos (SAA), TAC's major goal is to build a sunscreen development factory in Arusha, in order to provide adequate supplies of sunscreen to the tens of thousands of albinos living in Africa. TAC has also partnered with Assisting Children in Need (ACN), which will help the organization expand its dormitory to house more than 80 albino children, and another Dutch group, Cordaid, which provides educational funding for 38 albino children in Moshi and Kilimanjaro. In addition, TAC will soon establish a mobile health care clinic to serve the more than 800 albinos living in Arusha.[24]

The International Federation of Red Cross (IFRC) and Red Crescent Societies has collected food, clothes, cash, mattresses, and beds in Burundi in an attempt to reintegrate displaced albinos back into mainstream society, while simultaneously striving to minimize their vulnerability to hunters, skin cancer, and educational and social marginalization.[6] The IFRC has also established several institutions for displaced albinos, such as the Kabanga School for the Disabled in Kasulu, Tanzania, which offers shelter and protection for more than 50 albino children and their mothers who fled their homes in fear of persecution. However, the school is in dire need of support and improvement as it lacks a proper kitchen, dining hall, and beds to accommodate the increasing number of albinos who are attracted to the school as a safe haven from harassment. Bartha Ismaeli, a 15-year-old with albinism and her 3 albino siblings recently relocated to the school after hearing about albino killings on the radio, stating, "We were frightened that attackers might come for us.[25] When we are here, we feel

much safer. There is a day guard who watches us and, at night, two armed policemen come and count us before we enter the dorms. They then patrol the compound at night and that is how we know we are safe."[25]

Asante Mariamu, an organization named after Mariamu Staford, a Tanzanian woman with albinism who survived an attack by albino hunters, coupled with the word "asante," which means thank you in Swahili,[26] is determined to help stop the slaughter of albinos in East Africa, ensure swift prosecution and conviction of their killers, and provide life-saving education and supplies for skin cancer prevention. Positive Exposure, a project initiated by photographers Rick Guidotti and Diane McLean in 1997, portrays individuals with albinism in a positive light via photography and video clips. Positive Exposure also hosts self-esteem and self-advocacy workshops for albinos.[27]

The World Health Organization recently recognized albinism as a significant public health issue in sub-Saharan Africa[1] and has also established the WHO INTERSUN program,[28] which provides information about the adverse effects of UVR, stressing that overexposure can injure the skin, eyes, and immune system. Other albinism awareness groups in Africa and around the world that deserve recognition include the Albino Association of Malawi (TAAW), Tanzania Vision Support, and the National Organization for Albinism and Hypopigmentation (NOAH),[29] which is currently sponsoring a campaign to stop albino murders in East Africa, and various other support groups (see **Table 1**).

Albinism awareness and stories of persecution have also recently received international attention in media outlets such as the New York Times[30] and British Broadcasting Corporation (BBC), highlighting tragic stories such as that of a man who was caught attempting to sell his albino wife for about $3000[31] and 2 mothers who were hacked with machetes by gangs who were after their albino children.[32] Because of this persistent persecution, many albinos have opted to hide out in secluded rural areas, often separated from their friends and families.[30] Furthermore, since 2007, there have been more than 60 albino murders in Tanzania and Burundi, although conviction rates have been low. In 2009, 3 men were sentenced to hanging for the murder of an albino boy, a landmark case that represented the first ever conviction for albino murder.[33]

In early 2010, US Congressman Gerald Connelly, a democrat from Virginia, issued a statement urging President Barack Obama's participation in the fight against unwarranted albino killings in

Africa.[34,35] Connolly was inspired to propose the legislation following his meeting with Mariamu Staford a young albino woman from rural Tanzania who had both of her arms hacked off by fellow villagers, and whose story also inspired the formation of the Asante Mariamu organization by Susan and Doug DuBois. Connolly was further alarmed to learn that although Staford was able to identify the attackers, they had not been charged or arrested. During his proposal, Connolly stated that he "… applauded the dedicated group of local residents who brought Mariamu's story and the stories of other atrocities against people with albinism in East Africa to my attention. With their help and the passage of this resolution today, maybe we can bring an end to these horrific and heinous crimes,"[34] adding, "Tanzanian Prime Minister Mizengo Pinda has condemned the violent crimes against people with albinism, but judicial and enforcement barriers remain."[35]

The law, which urges local African governments to take immediate action to condemn the violence against albinos and persecute perpetrators, was passed by the House of Representatives on March 9, 2010, with an almost unanimous vote of 418 to 1.[34] Mariamu has since returned to the United States to be fitted with artificial arms.[35] The members of the European Union have also recently adopted a special resolution condemning the albino murders in Tanzania and Burundi and supporting justice for the victims and criminals.[35] In July 2010, the fourth National Conference on Albinism was held in Sokoto, Nigeria, to establish an international intervention for albinos living in Africa, with a central theme emphasizing that albinos may live free of skin cancer and persecution.[36]

PROPOSED SOLUTIONS

In 1990, Christianson and colleagues[37] initiated a clinical genetic outreach program in northern South Africa in which a network of genetic nurses was established to identify albino babies and offer immediate counseling and support. Lund[3] demonstrated that genetic care programs used in Northern Africa facilitated low-cost care, improved self-esteem, and increased community awareness. Today, in northern South Africa, pamphlets on albinism are available in various languages and genetic nurses often speak on the radio to raise awareness.[3] However, the usefulness of these pamphlets has been questioned, as albinos attending an outreach clinic in Tanzania did not have a better understanding of sun avoidance after reading the booklets.[9]

Unfortunately, awareness does not always lead to understanding, as Lund and Taylor[38] recently demonstrated at a special school for visually impaired children in South Africa. Although most children possessed hats, the brim widths were found to be insufficient in terms of face and neck protection, resulting in visible sun damage. The average brim width was 5.4 cm, far narrower than the minimum of 7.5 cm suggested by Diffey and Cheeseman[39] after their studies with model head forms and ultraviolet-sensitive film badges. Although the students understood the need to use sunscreen, they did not understand the term SPF (sun protection factor) and only applied the lotion sporadically; one-third were not wearing it at the time of interview.[38] Many students did not apply sunscreen every day, instead rationing their limited supply to last as long as possible.[38] Thus, even at a private boarding school for children with visual impairments, where more education on albinism and sun protection strategies was provided, albinism understanding was not universal, prompting the need for improved teaching techniques.

Lund and Gaigher[15] have suggested a team approach including children, teachers, parents, health officials, and the wider community. Lund and Taylor[37] have also suggested using individuals with albinism to deliver information about sun protection and initiate support groups to provide firsthand knowledge about their experiences to individuals with a similar condition. The public must be informed that apart from a genetically induced lack of pigment, albinos are normal human beings. In particular, public school teachers should be aware of their eye problems and make proper provisions in the classroom, such as permitting them to sit close to the blackboard. Albinism is not associated with abnormal intelligence, but this is a common belief among educators, likely because of poor vision and the resultant setbacks at school. Other suggestions include enlarged textbooks and provision of magnifying lenses.[22] Albinos must be educated about the cause of their condition and the implications of marrying a relative with regular pigmentation. Although most albinos have albino relatives, most of them are not aware that their condition is inherited. And perhaps most importantly, the IFRC suggests that, "the first step in the response to the aftermath of the killings, as with any humanitarian intervention, is to register the beneficiaries. But in this 'silent emergency' they must first be found. In the current atmosphere of mortal danger, albinos in remote rural areas (still the vast majority) are only likely to reveal themselves to community-based Red Cross volunteers."[6]

SUMMARY

Although there is currently no cure for albinism, many of the associated morbidities can be prevented with improved security, proper sun protection, and eye care. In Africa, sunscreen is costly and difficult to attain, and many believe that the solution is UVR avoidance and protective outerwear, which can be achieved with community-wide education and distribution of sun-shielding garments.[3] To better meet the many medical and psychosocial needs of individuals with albinism in Africa, awareness groups and public health interventions must continue to gain support. Society as a whole must become aware that stigmas and negative attitudes have a significant effect on the social, emotional, and psychological aspect of an albino's quality of life.

ACKNOWLEDGMENTS

The authors kindly acknowledge Dorothy Shope for the contribution of photographs and Mariya Mazuryan JD for her editorial efforts.

REFERENCES

1. Hong ES, Zeeb H, Repacholi MH. Albinism in Africa as a public health issue. BMC Public Health 2006;6:212.
2. Simona BE. Albinos in black Africa. Int J Dermatol 2004;43:618–21.
3. Lund PM. Oculocutaneous albinism in southern Africa. Ann Hum Biol 2005;32(2):168–73.
4. Witkop CJ, Quevedo WC, Fitzpatrick TB, et al. Albinism. The metabolic basis of inherited disease. New York: McGraw-Hill; 1989. p. 2905–2947.
5. Braun-Falco O, Plewig G, Wolff HH. Dermatologie und Venerologie. Germany: Ludwig Maximilian Universitat Munchen, Klinik fur Dermatologie und Venerologie der Medizinischen Universitat Lubeck; 2006.
6. International Federation of Red Cross (IFRC) and Red Crescent Societies. Through albino eyes. The plight of albino people in Africa's Great Lake's region and a Red Cross response. Advocacy Report. 2009.
7. Aquaron R, Djatou M, Kamdem L. [Sociocultural aspects of albinism in sub-Saharan Africa: mutilations and ritual murders committed in East Africa (Burundi and Tanzania)]. Med Trop (Mars) 2009 Oct;69(5):449–53 [in French].
8. Okema M. Apartheid in reverse: the fate of albinos. The East African 1999.
9. McBride SR, Leppard BJ. Attitudes and beliefs of an albino population toward sun avoidance. Arch Dermatol 2002;138:629–32.
10. Kuster R. White skin, black souls. New African 2000;382:40–1.
11. Kromberg JGR, Zwaine EM, Jenkins T. The response of black mothers to the birth of an albino infant. Am J Dis Child 1987;141:911–6.
12. Kromberg JGR. Albinism in South Africa negro: IV. Attitudes and the death myth. Birth Defects 1992; 28:159–66.
13. Kromberg JGR, Castle D, Zwane EM, et al. Albinism and skin cancer in southern Africa. Clin Genet 1989; 36:43–52.
14. Lund PM. Distribution of oculocutaneous albinism in Zimbabwe. J Med Genet 1996;33:641–4.
15. Lund PM, Gaigher R. A health intervention programme for children with albinism at a special school in South Africa. Health Educ Res 2002;17:365–72.
16. Lund PM. Health and education of children with albinism in Zimbabwe. Health Educ Res 2001; 16:1–7.
17. Okoro AN. Albinism in Nigeria: a clinical and social study. Br J Dermatol 1975;92:485–92.
18. King RA, Creel D, Cervenka J, et al. Albinism in Nigeria with delineation of new recessive oculocutaneous type. Clin Genet 1980;17:259–70.
19. Luande J, Henschke CI, Mohammed N. The Tanzanian human albino skin. Cancer 1985;55:1823–8.
20. Kagore F, Pm Lund. Oculocutaneous albinism among schoolchildren in Harare, Zimbabwe. J Med Genet 1995;32:859–61.
21. Gaigher RJ, Lund PM, Makuya E. A sociological study of children with albinism at a special school in the Limpopo province. Curationis 2002;25:4–11.
22. Simona B. Regional dermatological training center. Int J Dermatol 2004;43(8):618–21.
23. Manier J. More than skin deep. University of Chicago Magazine; 2010. Available at: http://magazine. uchicago.edu/0906/chicago_journal/onthemap. shtml. Accessed July 1, 2010.
24. Tanzania Albino Centre. Available at: http://www.tanzaniaalbino.org. Accessed July 1, 2010.
25. Wanjiru A. Tanzanian albinos face deplorable living conditions in safe haven. Available at: http://www. ifrc.org/docs/news/10/10053102/index.asp. Accessed May 31, 2010.
26. Asante Mariamu. Available at: www.asante-mariamu.org. Accessed July 1, 2010.
27. Positive Exposure. Available at: www.positiveexposure.org. Accessed July 1, 2010.
28. WHO Intersun Programme. World Health Organization. Available at: http://www.who.int/uv. Accessed July 1, 2010.
29. National Organization for Albinism and Hypopigmentation (NOAH). Available at: http://www.albinism. org/faq/pwa.html. Accessed July 1, 2010.
30. Gettleman J. Albinos, long shunned, face threat in Tanzania. New York Times; 2008. Available at: http://www.nytimes.com/2008/06/08/world/africa/08albino. html?pagewanted=1. Accessed July 3, 2010.

31. BBC News. Man 'tried to sell' albino wife 2008. Available at: http://news.bbc.co.uk/2/hi/africa/7726743.stm. Accessed July 3, 2010.

32. BBC News. Mothers hacked in albino attacks 2008. Available at: http://news.bbc.co.uk/2/hi/africa/7730193.stm. Accessed July 3, 2010.

33. Howden D. Three sentenced to hang for murder of an African 'ghost'. The Independent 2009. Available at: http://www.independent.co.uk/news/world/africa/three-sentenced-to-hang-for-murder-of-an-african-ghost-1792295.html. Accessed July 3, 2010.

34. ThisDay Reporter. US Congress passes new law against albinos torture, killings. This Day 2010. Available at: http://www.thisday.co.tz/?l=10722. Accessed July 5, 2010.

35. NGO News Africa. Tanzania: albino killings - Obama asked to put pressure on Kikwete 2010. Available at: http://www.ngonewsafrica.org/2010/02/tanzania-albino-killings-obama-asked-to.html. Accessed July 5, 2010.

36. Afrique Avenir. Nigeria to host conference on albinism intervention in Africa 2010. Available at: http://www.afriqueavenir.org/en/2010/07/11/nigeria-to-host-conference-on-albinism-intervention-in-africa. Accessed July 31, 2010.

37. Christianson AL, Venter PA, Modiba JH, et al. Development of a primary health care clinical genetic service in rural South Africa—the northern province experience, 1990–1996. Community Genet 2000;3:77–84.

38. Lund PM, Taylor JS. Lack of adequate sun protection for children with oculocutaneous albinism in South Africa. BMC Public Health 2008;8:225.

39. Diffey BL, Cheeseman J. Sun protection with hats. Br J Dermatol 1992;127(1):10–2.

Innate Immunity and *Leishmania* Vaccination Strategies

Ron Birnbaum, MD[a], Noah Craft, MD, PhD, DTM&H[a,b],*

KEYWORDS

- Cutaneous leishmaniasis • Vaccine • Immunotherapy
- *Leishmania* • Toll-like receptors • Innate immunity

THE PROBLEM OF VACCINES FOR PARASITES: CUTANEOUS LEISHMANIASIS AS AN EXAMPLE

Despite advances in understanding of their epidemiology, vector ecology, disease pathogenesis, and treatments, parasites continue to ravage humanity. Unlike many viral and bacterial illnesses, there remain no effective and safe vaccines for parasitic illness in widespread use. The economics of private sector drug and vaccine development likely contribute to the relative neglect of parasitic diseases. Increased attention to these neglected tropical diseases in the public and nonprofit sectors has also not yet led to parasite vaccines. Technical challenges and the complexity of immunity to parasites clearly contribute to the absence of vaccines. The history of attempts to vaccinate against cutaneous leishmaniasis may be 1000 years old. Progress, controversy, and challenges in *Leishmania* vaccination have been reviewed previously.[1–7] In this review, we examine the specific role that innate immunity plays in past and future leishmania vaccination strategies.

OVERVIEW OF VACCINE USEFULNESS FOR LEISHMANIASIS

The leishmaniases are heterogeneous diseases of the developing world caused by infection with unicellular protozoan parasites of the genus *Leishmania* and transmitted by the bite of an infected phlebotomine sand fly.[8] Ingested *Leishmania* develop in the gut of sand flies in the promastigote (flagellated) stage and are regurgitated on subsequent bites along with immunoactive elements of fly saliva. Promastigotes infect mammalian hosts' innate immune cells, primarily macrophages in the skin. Within macrophage phagosomes, *Leishmania* assume the amastigote (round, nonflagellated) form and proliferate. In cutaneous leishmaniasis (eg, infection with *Leishmania major*), macrophage infection results in either subclinical infection or subacute to chronic disease characterized by skin ulceration and scarring. Progressive spread to destructive mucosal leishmaniasis (ML) can occur in some individuals.[9] In visceral leishmaniasis (VL), typified by disease caused by *Leishmania donovani* or *Leishmania chagasi/infantum*, parasites disseminate to the

Support and potential conflicts of interest: no financial support. There are no identifiable conflicts of interest. Other potential conflicts of interest: NC has received research funding from Graceway Pharmaceuticals {Zimmermann, 2008 #3611} and 3M Pharmaceuticals. NC and RB are coinventors on patent applications covering the use of Killed But Metabolically Active protozoan vaccines and the use of Toll-like receptor agonists as adjuvants with these vaccines.

[a] Los Angeles Biomedical Research Institute at Harbor-UCLA Medical Center, LA BioMed, Building HH-207, 1124 West Carson Street, Torrance, CA 90502, USA

[b] David Geffen School of Medicine at the University of California, Los Angeles, 10833 Le Conte Avenue, Los Angeles, CA 90095, USA

* Corresponding author. LA BioMed, Building HH-207, 1124 West Carson Street, Torrance, CA 90502.
E-mail address: ncraft@ucla.edu

Dermatol Clin 29 (2011) 89–102
doi:10.1016/j.det.2010.08.014

spleen, liver, and bone marrow, resulting in subclinical clearance of the parasite or parasitemia and eventual death. Leishmaniasis presents an onerous disease burden in endemic areas in South and Central America, Africa, the Middle East, and south Asia. Annually, 2 million humans are infected with *Leishmania* spp and 70,000 die from leishmaniasis.[8] Morbidity from nonlethal cases includes disfigurement and disability. Treatments, including antimonial compounds and amphotericin, are only variably effective, toxic, and expensive.[4,8,10] Efforts to develop vaccines against leishmaniasis for humans are justified by the following concepts: (1) prevalence of and morbidity/mortality associated with infections; (2) cost, toxicity, and ineffectiveness of current treatments; (3) natural infection in humans frequently leads to durable immunity; (4) demonstrable efficacy of experimental vaccines in various animal models; and (5) in some cases (primarily VL) leishmaniases are, like smallpox, anthroponotic infections and thus vaccination holds hope for complete eradication of the disease.

IMMUNITY TO *LEISHMANIA*
Basic Host Mechanisms

Host factors such as age, nutritional status, pregnancy, and human immunodeficiency virus (HIV) infection[11] contribute to varied disease severity, but many infected persons develop subclinical infections. These facts underscore the importance of host immunity to disease pathogenesis. With cutaneous leishmaniasis, humans who clear an initial infection, either spontaneously or with medical therapy, normally have lifelong immunity to that species. Additionally, in both cutaneous and VL, after a subclinical infection many humans in endemic areas develop lasting immunity, as manifest by conversion to leishmanin skin test positivity. The central irony of leishmaniasis is that the macrophage is both the principal immune effector cell charged with killing *Leishmania* amastigotes and also the principal site of parasite proliferation and dissemination. Resolution of infection with *Leishmania* is associated with presentation of *Leishmania* antigens by macrophages and dendritic cells (DCs) and priming of CD4 and CD8 lymphocytes. Ultimately, induction of nitric oxide synthase (iNOS) and interferon-γ (IFN-γ) leads to macrophage nitric oxide (NO) production, reactive oxygen species (ROS), and parasite killing.[12,13] Recent evidence supports the contention that sustained immunity may require persistent low-level infection with parasites.[12,14,15] *Leishmania* infection may be modulated at several time points including control of the initial infection by innate immune cells (neutrophils, natural killer

[NK] cells, mast cells, and macrophages) or during development of lasting immunity (characterized by central memory and effector T cells). The role of B cells in early control of parasite load and in the progress toward adaptive immunity as antigen-presenting cells (APC) has received increasing attention lately. The role of Toll-like receptors (TLRs) in this pathway may also be important.[16] There are many proposed mechanisms for *Leishmania* eluding effector mechanisms of the immune system:

1. Inhibition of macrophage phagosomal killing functions, both NO and ROS mediated
2. Inhibition of macrophage phagosomal maturation (interfering with fusion of phagosomes and lysozomes)[12]
3. Inhibition of DC maturation and chemotaxis[17]
4. Recruitment of inhibitory CD4$^+$CD25$^+$FoxP3$^+$ regulatory T cells (T-regs)[12,14,18]
5. Biasing the immune program away from the effective cellular response (coordinated by Th1-type CD4$^+$ helper T cells in association with interleukin (IL)-12 and IFN-γ) and toward the ineffective humoral/antihelminthic response (typified by Th2-type CD4$^+$ helper T cells in association with IL-4, IL-5, and IL-13).[12,13,19--21] A governing principle in *Leishmania* vaccinology is that successful immunity to *Leishmania* requires establishment of a Th1-dominated cell-mediated adaptive immune response.[22]

In addition to natural T-regs that express FoxP3, other regulatory T cell subsets that secrete IL-10 and/or TGF-β have been implicated in chronic or nonhealing disease states in both animal models and human disease.[12,21] IL-10 is notable because of its direct suppressive effect on phagocyte/APC function. Some investigators have proposed a dynamic equilibrium state of persistent low-level infection that serves as a perpetual reservoir for protective antigenic stimulation of the host but that places the host at risk for later recrudescence,[12,14,23] especially in the context of the immunosuppression of HIV disease. Using what is known about the fundamental mechanisms of natural immunity to leishmaniasis as a scaffold, this article reviews vaccine strategy and the role of innate immunity in these strategies.

Th1-Th2 Paradigm and the Role Innate Immunity Plays in Th1-Th2 Polarization

Animal models instruct studies on the immunopathogenesis of leishmaniasis and vaccine development. T cell deficient mice suffer overwhelming infection with various *Leishmania* species. This susceptibility can be reversed with the adoptive transfer of normal T cells.[7] C57BL/6 mice infected with *L major* develop a type 1 (Th1) immune response and resist infection. BALB/c mice develop a type 2 (Th2) immune response and chronic progressive infection. This observation was the first demonstration of relationship between Th1/Th2 responses and an infectious disease outcome in a mammalian model.[7,13,19–21] Mice rendered deficient in specific proteins either by genetic or antibody-mediated elimination have refined this view, showing the centrality of specific cytokines including IFN-γ, IL-4, IL-10, and IL-12, in protection.[12] Because of their susceptibility to progressive chronic *Leishmania* infection, BALB/c mice remain an important model for both visceral and cutaneous disease; C57BL/6 mice remain important models for disease resistance and its determinants. Although the Th1/Th2 dichotomy remains the governing dogma in *Leishmania* immunity, important contravening examples exist. For example, the Syrian hamster is considered by some to be a more representative model to study the progressive side of human disease because, despite the Th1-type immune response of the hamster, they ultimately develop progressive disease because of reduced iNOS ativity.[24] The role of iNOS induction in this model has been a central area of research. In humans, it is not the group of patients with strong and effective adaptive immune responses that needs help. People with robust but ineffective humoral responses are the ones who must be protected or treated more aggressively. One approach is to focus attention on manipulations of the innate immune system to ultimately induce an effective and protective durable immunity.

Persistent Parasites After Clinical Resolution

Resistant C57BL/6 mice seem to resolve infection and then develop sustained resistance to subsequent infections. However, careful studies have shown that apparently resolved infections involved the low-level presence of persistent parasites[12,14,23] at the site of initial infection and draining lymph nodes. This population of parasites may be sustained by a state of dynamic equilibrium between the parasitogenic Th1 effects and the immunoinhibitory effects of antigen-specific T-regs and IL-10. Sterile resolution of infections may be associated with eventual loss of lasting immunity. Thus, the notion of memory in *Leishmania* infection could be reconceived as frequent reminders from ongoing presence of antigen. Reactivation of leishmaniasis (in scars or at sites of old infections) is common in the context of certain conditions like

acquired immune deficiency syndrome and with waning immunity caused by advanced age.[11]

Nevertheless, recent studies in mice show an unequivocal role for lymphocytes with memory phenotype in resistance to leishmaniasis. The CD4$^+$ T cells responsible for immunity to *L major* included 2 populations: effector T cells that home to tissues, produce cytokines, and require persistent parasites for survival, and central memory T cells (Tcm) that home to lymph nodes, express molecules such as CCR7 and CD62L, and persist in the absence of parasites.[25,26] Transfer of either of these populations from immunized mice affords protection to donor mice from virulent challenge. Significantly, no role has been described for effector memory T cells (Tem) in durable immunity. Thus, the established model for durable immunity in the absence of parasite persistence involves antigen-specific Tcm cells that can quickly proliferate and differentiate into tissue-homing, IFN-γ–producing effector cells. By implication, any vaccine strategy that does not depend on live virulent parasites must have as one of its aims the generation of an antigen-specific Tcm cell population. The role of the innate immune system in establishing Tcm or Tem remains undefined. However, manipulation of the innate immune system with a vaccine (eg, by potent adjuvants or other mechanisms) could potentially alter the equilibrium in strategies that require persistent parasites (eg, by being too successful in complete parasite elimination). Alternatively, strong adjuvants, in theory, could contribute positively to the establishment of durable immunity in the absence of persistence parasites. The need for persistent parasites and the risks associated with them will remain key issues in *Leishmania* vaccination strategies. This concept would encourage the use of live vaccines that are attenuated genetically or otherwise.[2,6]

ROLE OF THE INNATE IMMUNE SYSTEM IN NATURAL AND VACCINE-INDUCED IMMUNITY

The role of adaptive immunity (ie, antigen-specific T and B cell responses associated with immunologic memory, especially specific CD4+ and CD8+ T cell responses) is well established in *Leishmania* studies. The innate immune system consists of fungible cells of hematopoietic lineage (ie, macrophages, DCs, NK cells, neutrophils, eosinophils, and mast cells) that play a variety of roles as phagocytes, pathogen killers, antigen-presenting cells, and producers of biochemical signals. These cells characteristically do not display long-term antigen-specific memory behavior. However, they do participate in the specificity of the immune response via the mechanism of pattern recognition receptors (PRR) that recognize stereotypical biochemical motifs on foreign organisms and identify those as nonself and potentially dangerous. The TLR family is typical of PRRs and highly relevant to immunity against *Leishmania* and other parasites. The innate immune system also includes a variety of soluble antimicrobial entities (including antimicrobial peptides and the protein components of the complement system) and PRR on adaptive immune cells and nonhematopoietic cells. The skin itself participates in innate immunity as a mechanical barrier to infections, although no specific evidence suggests that skin barrier compromise facilitates infections with *Leishmania*. The innate immune system is reviewed in **Table 1** and a limited summary of roles of relevant innate immune cell types is provided. **Table 2** provides a summary of known roles of PRR and other molecular elements of the innate immune system in *Leishmania* resistance.

Cells of the innate immune system recognize conserved components of microbial pathogens called pathogen-associated molecular patterns (PAMPs)[25] via PRR.[27–30] Besides TLRs, other examples of PRRs include intracellular NOD-like receptors,[29–31] and scavenger receptors.[32] Activation of TLRs by PAMPs leads to inflammatory cytokine production and a characteristic antimicrobial immune responses by innate immune cells such as macrophages, DC, NK cells, and granulocytes.[27–29,33]

Increasing numbers of studies show that TLRs are important in host defense against bacteria and other microbial pathogens.[28,29] So far, 11 members (TLR1–TLR11) have been described in mouse and human genomes. These members are activated by different microbial components including bacterial peptidoglycan and lipoproteins, triacyl and diacyl lipopeptides, virus-derived double-stranded RNA (dsRNA), bacterial endotoxin (eg, lipopolysaccharide [LPS]), bacterial flagellin, unmethylated DNA sequences (CpG motifs) found in bacterial DNA,[28,29] and single-stranded RNA (ssRNA).[34] Both ssRNA and the imadazoquinoline family of synthetic small molecules activate TLR7 and TLR8.[35] Lipophosphoglycans (LPG) on the *Leishmania* cell surface have been implicated as agonists of TLR2[36] and have also been associated with NK cell activation in *L major* infection.[17] Stimulation of TLRs ultimately results in gene expression profiles that lead to the production of cytokines including TNF-α, IL-1, IL-6, and IL-12, as well as type I interferons (IFN-α and IFN-β).[29,37] Many TLRs, including TLR2, TLR4, TLR7, TLR8, and TLR9, transduce intracellular signals through the adaptor molecule MyD88. This cascade ultimately leads to NF-kB/AP1 activation and transcription of genes encoding proinflammatory cytokines and chemokines.[35] Mice defective in MyD88 are highly susceptible to *Leishmania* infection, implicating this pathway in antileishmanial immunity.[36,38,39] The susceptibility of MyD88-deficient C57BL/6 mice to *L major* infection is associated with a pathologic Th2-dominated response that reverts to a wild-type Th1-dominated phenotype by addition of exogenous IL-12.[39]

Although the role of TLR in natural immunity to *Leishmania* and in vaccine strategies have been investigated with increasing interest, questions about their significance remain. By contrast, no published studies report any investigation into the function of NODs in *Leishmania*, although the relevance of NOD1 to immunity to *Trypanosoma cruzi* provides a tantalizing invitation to investigators interested in this possibility.

CURRENT APPROACHES TO *LEISHMANIA* VACCINES

Because of the unquestionable role of the immune system in controlling *Leishmania* infection, vaccination remains an attractive disease prevention strategy. Furthermore, although in some areas zoonotic reservoirs for certain species clearly exist, in others, the disease is considered anthroponotic, and thus targeted vaccination campaigns hold the hope for disease eradication as achieved with smallpox vaccination.[8] Armed with an appreciation of the pervasiveness of innate immune effector cells and molecules, this article discusses the strategies behind vaccines that have been investigated, tried, and proposed through the specific lens of innate immunity. *Leishmania* vaccines can be divided into 4 main groups: vaccination with live virulent parasites (termed leishmanization); vaccination with killed parasites (first-generation vaccines); vaccination with subunits, purified fractions, recombinant vaccines in heterologous microbial vectors, and genetically or otherwise attenuated live parasites (second-generation vaccines); and DNA-based vaccines (third-generation vaccines). Adjuvants have played a role in nearly every strategy, as detailed later. A brief history of *Leishmania* vaccine attempts could be summarized as follows: leishmanization works but is not acceptably safe and is difficult to standardize. Killed vaccines have proven safe but not effective in preventing infections. Subsequently, investigators have sought to develop a vaccine as effective as leishmanization and as safe as killed vaccines. Although the safety difference between these vaccines is easy to comprehend, the efficacy difference is not obvious; the chasm between the efficacy of live and killed vaccines is explored in this review.

The long-standing practice of leishmanization in certain endemic areas involves the inoculation of live *L major* parasites (generally without adjuvants) in the skin of children in cosmetically hidden areas such as the buttocks. The goal is to induce a mild infection and subsequent immunity,[8,40–42] but the practice has been largely abandoned as unsafe. Heat-killed or autoclaved *Leishmania* vaccines for cutaneous leishmaniasis have been in field trials since the 1940s in Brazil and more recently in Asia and Africa. Most of these studies used bacille Calmette-Guérin (BCG) as adjuvant. A recent meta-analysis of these studies[43] reports neither protection nor increased risk. Only a single study of the 11 reviewed (from Ecuador) showed statistically significant protection. What can account for the difference in efficacy between live whole-cell and heat-killed vaccines? We offer 6 different possibilities or models for the difference:

1. The inactivation process destroys antigen epitopes relevant to establishing protective adaptive responses.[43]
2. The inactivation process may destroy PAMPs, leading to inadequate activation of PRR in hosts and loss of key contributions to innate immunity.
3. The inactivation process produces or exposes new molecular determinants that are themselves immunoinhibitory. For example, the curious observation that *Leishmania* shows preserved programs for apoptosis raises the question, why would a unicellular organism need programmed cell death? A proposed answer has been that phagocytosed apoptotic parasites may suppress macrophage function in a manner similar to the way apoptotic neutrophils and other host cells have also been shown to suppress macrophage function.[26] In our hands, both live and metabolically active but replication-incompetent parasites induce bone marrow–derived macrophages to produce excess NO in the presence of IFN-γ. However, heat-killed parasites fail to have this effect (Birnbaum R and Craft N, unpublished data, 2010).
4. The inactivation process eliminates the metabolic activity of parasites. Absent byproducts of metabolism or the diminished consumption of substrates eliminates one or more signals that prompt host immunity.
5. Replication activity of live parasites could produce signals that stimulate protective immune responses. For example, if amastigote

replication proceeds unchecked in a macrophage and ends with the lytic death of that macrophage, the elaboration of intracellular host factors from this unnatural death process could provide crucial cues to the immune system. This notion follows the Danger Hypothesis advanced by Matzinger.[44] Host signals with immunomodulatory effects of this sort have been termed alarmins or danger-associated molecular patterns (DAMPs).[45]

6. Persistent parasites may be necessary for ongoing protection and would be absent in inactivated vaccines.

Additional vaccination strategies in humans have included heat-killed and parasite subunit vaccination along with adjuvants such as BCG.[17,46–49] Both preventive and therapeutic vaccinations have been attempted. Animal models have used a broader array of subunits and adjuvants. Past experience with vaccination in humans supports a special role for the immunogenicity of viable organisms, but is limited by risks and difficulties in standardization of whole-cell vaccines. Because the status of existing vaccines has been recently reviewed extensively,[1–7] we have focused more here on the conceptual role of the innate immune system in current and future vaccines.

EMPHASIS ON THE ROLE OF THE INNATE IMMUNE SYSTEM

Imiquimod is an immunomodulatory, small-molecule compound in the imidazoquinoline family that displays both antiviral and antitumor effects.[50,51] Imiquimod has primarily TLR7 activity in mice and in humans.[52] Approved for the treatment of genital warts, basal cell carcinoma, and actinic keratoses, imiquimod has been used clinically for an increasingly wide range of infectious and neoplastic skin disorders. Topical treatment with imiquimod induces a variety of proinflammatory cytokines including IFN-α, TNF-α, and IL-12,[53–55] and facilitates the maturation and migratory capabilities of DCs.[56] Resiquimod is a potent congener imidazoquinioline that also activates human and murine TLR7 and also human (but not murine) TLR8.[52] TLR7 agonists can synergize with the CD40 ligand to stimulate CD8$^+$ T cell responses and can selectively induce IL-12 and TNF-α from CD11c$^+$, CD11b$^+$, CD8$^-$ DCs.[57] In other vaccine studies, imidazoquinoline TLR agonists have been shown to redirect immune responses toward the Th1 type, as shown by cytokine and antibody isotype profiling.[58] In the setting of established tolerance, recent evidence

Table 1
Review of roles of innate immune system cells in anti-leishmanial immunity

Innate Immune Cell Type	Identified Roles
Neutrophils	Most immediate responder[67,68]
	Kill promastigotes via reactive oxygen and reactive nitrogen species as well as neutrophil extracellular traps[69]
	Highly stimulated by sand fly saliva even in absence or presence of parasites[70]
	May facilitate parasitization of macrophages (but not DCs) via either Trojan horse or other mechanisms[68]
	Apoptotic neutrophils at infection site may suppress macrophage function[70]
	Beneficial role in C57BL/6 (resistant) mice L major infection, associated with upregulated TLR2,TLR7,TLR9, IL-12p70, and IL-10[71]
	Pathologic role in BALB/C (susceptible) mice L major infection, associated with immunoinhibitory IL-12p40 homodimers[71]
	Beneficial role in BALB/c mice infected with L brazilensis[72]
	Limit efficacy of killed L major vaccine in C57BL/6 mice[73]
Macrophages	Definitive host cell dwelling and replication site for amastigotes
	Definitive pathogen killer via NO mediated by synergistic effect of IFN-γ and TNF-α
	Phagocytose Leishmania spp via mannose receptor, complement receptors 1 and 3, TLR2, and TLR3.[74]
	L major GP63 surface protease leads to activation of macrophage protein tyrosine phosphatases (like SHP-1), and suppression of macrophage activation and killing function[75]
	Classic macrophage activation: increased iNOS activity and NO, decreased urea production: parasite killing[76,77]
	Alternative macrophage activation: decreased iNOS2 activity, increased arginase 1 activity, associated with Th2 response and poor healing[76,77]
	L major—associated arginase enhances parasite replication and disease pathogenesis in BALB/c mice[78]

Cell	
DCs	May be the key cell that mediates the innate immune system's instructive role on Th1 vs Th2 fate via antigen presentation to and priming of specific CD4 helper T cell subsets and NK cells[79–81]
	Produce IL-12 (vital for Th1 development) in response to *Leishmania* spp uptake in manner that is dependent on MyD88, the adapter protein critical to most TLR signaling[82]
	Migratory dermal DCs part of early uptake of *Leishmania*[83]
	Detect *Leishmania* phosphoglycans (such as lipophosphoglycans) with complex effects on Th1 vsTh2 responses[84]
	Integrate signals from PRR including TLR2, 3, 4, 7, 9 resulting in cytokine release and direct Th helper subset polarity such as Th1, Th2, Th17[79,80,85]
	DCs with capacity to protect mice from *Leishmania* may direct Th1 vs Th2 polarization in *Leishmania* infection by expression of specific Notch-family ligands[86]
	Leishmania spp actively downmodulate DC cytokine production[79,85]
	iNOS-producing DC are the major infected cell type in the chronic phase of parasite persistence in C57BL/6 *L major* infection[87]
NK cells	*L major* lipophosphoglycans upregulate TLR2 in human NK cells resulting in increased IFN-γ, TNF-α, and NF-κB nuclear translocation[88]
	Human NK secrete IFN-γ directly in response to live, but not killed, *Leishmania* promastigote stimulation or to stimulation with *Leishmania pifanoi* amastigote antigen P-2 (a cysteine proteinase)[89,90]
	Activated by DC in vaccine condition with TLR9 agonists C57BL/6 mice[81]
	NK cells activate *L donovani* infected allogeneic BALB/c mouse macrophages via TNF-α but not IFN-γ. These activated NK are not cytotoxic against promastigotes or infected macrophages[91]
Mast cells	Mediate resistance to infection in C57BL/6 mice to *L major* via recruitment of neutrophils, macrophages, and DCs and via increased IL-12production and favorable Th1 immune response, and TLR2 expression.[92,93]
	Early degranulation of mast cells contributes to susceptibility of BALB/c mice in *L major* and *L mexicana* infection.[93,94]

Table 2
Summary of known roles of PRR and other molecular elements of the innate immune system in *Leishmania* resistance

Innate Immune Receptor Molecules	Identified Role
TLRs (in general)	*L major* infection induced TLR2, TLR4, TLR7, TLR9 (but not TLR1, TLR3, TLR5, TLR8) transcription in mouse neutrophil infection in BALB/C and C57BL/6 mice[71] TLR2, TLR 7, TLR9 (but not TLR4) showed significantly greater transcription in resistant C57BL/6 mouse neutrophils compared with susceptible BALB/C mice[71] MyD88 null mice show increased susceptibility to *Leishmania* infection. MyD88 is involved in some TLR signaling[95]
TLR2	Activated by *Leishmania* spp lipophosphoglycans, a confirmed TLR2 agonist that stimulates IFN-γ, TNF-α, and nuclear translocation of NF-κB on human NK cells[36,88] TLR2 plays a role in phagocytosis of *L donovani* promastigotes[74] *Lpg2*−/− *L major* that cannot synthesize lipophosphoglycans show attenuated pathogenicity but protective vaccine immunogenicity and maintain low-level infective persistence without inducing strong Th1 responses in BALB/C mice[96] Soluble lipophosphoglycans induces macrophage NO production and ROS production in macrophage cell lines, production of Th1 cytokines, and suppression of IL-10 in a TLR2 (but not TLR4)-dependent manner[82,97] TLR2 null mice are less susceptible to *L amazonensis* infection and show granulomalike eosinophilic nodules and diminished mononuclear and neutrophil infiltration in early infection of ear dermis of C57BL/6 mice[98] Has both MyD88-dependent and -independent signaling properties as MyD88 null mice show increased susceptibility to *Leishmania* infection, whereas TLR2 null mice show increased resistance (ie, TLR2 has an immunomodulatory effect on infection)[99]
TLR4	Activated in *L major* infection and associated with increase iNOS activity and decreased arginase activity (ie, classic as opposed to alternative macrophage activation). No known TLR4 ligand on *Leishmania* but in vivo effects may be mediated by endogenous host ligands such as heat shock proteins or extracellular matrix elements elaborated during infection[100] C57BL/10 mice null at TLR4 locus show a nonhealing phenotype to *L major* infection but not a shift from Th1 to Th2 response[100]
TLR7 and TLR8	Efficacy of TLR7 agonists imiquimod and TLR 7/8 resiquimod as immunotherapeutics and vaccine adjuvants in CL (mice and humans)[62] Efficacy of imiquimod and resiquimod as vaccine adjuvants and immunotherapeutic agents against *L chagasi* in mice (Birnbaum R and Craft N, unpublished data, 2010)

TLR9	Extensive use of bacterial CpG associated with TLR9 activation, Th1 polarization, and protection in prophylactic and therapeutic vaccines in mouse and primate models[23,63,64] *Leishmania* DNA may activate immune cells directly via TLR9[101]
Inducible iNOS	Produces leishmanicidal NO in DCs after *Leishmania* infection[87] Competes with arginase for substrate, arginine, which converts arginine into urea and orthinine; the latter is necessary for polyamine synthesis necessary for *Leishmania* growth[102] iNOS null c57BL/6 mice are susceptible to progressive infection with *L braziliensis* unlike C57BL/6 WT mice which are resistant[103]
C3	Rapidly lyses 95% of free promastigotes (human $\gg$ mouse) via alternative complement pathway (*L donovani* and *L amazonensis*)[104] Opsonization of *Leishmania* with C3a associated with phagocytosis (invasion) of macrophages via C3R[104] Mediates immune adherence to erythrocytes, which facilitates promastigote endocytosis and circumvents lysis[104] *Leishmania* parasite surface antigen 2 interacts with C3 to facilitate macrophage invasion[105] Upregulated by TLR9 agonists (CpG ODN)[106]
Suppressors of cytokine signaling family SOCS-1 and SOCS-3	Expression induced by *L major* lipophosphoglycan in macrophages. SOCS-1 is associated with modulation of IFN-γ effects[36]
MARCO	Non-TLR PRR of the scavenger receptor family Increased in *L major* but not *L amazonensis* infections[32] Plays role in *L major* infection of CBA/J mouse macrophages as anti-MARCO monoclonal Ab reduces *L major* macrophage infection 30%–40%[32]
Antimicrobial peptides	Broad range of direct activity and host immunomodulation[107]
Sand fly saliva components	Facilitate macrophage recruitment and alternative macrophage activation[108] Drive immunity toward protective response against *Leishmania*[109,110]

Abbreviations: C3, complement 3; MARCO, macrophage receptor with collagenous structure.

Table 3
Mechanisms used by *Leishmania* species to subvert the immune system

Leishmania Immune Pathogenesis	TLR7/8 Counteracting Effects
Macrophage phagosome maturation inhibition	Stimulates maturation
Macrophage killing inhibition	Stimulates killing via IFN-γ
DC maturation arrest	Stimulates DC activation/maturation
Th2 over Th1	Th1 stimulation
Induction of IL-10	Downregulates IL-10
Induction of T regulatory cells	Deactivation of T regulatory cells

suggests that persistent TLR signaling is required for bypassing regulatory T cell–induced tolerance.[38,59] Regulatory T cells have been shown to have important and complex roles in *Leishmania* immunity, especially in rendering the skin an area for immune privilege and thus a reservoir for ongoing and recurring infection.[12,14]

Several investigators have proposed the use of TLR agonists as topical therapeutics for cutaneous leishmaniasis[60,61] and as adjuvants for *Leishmania* prophylactic and therapeutic vaccines, particularly imidazoquinolines with TLR7 and TLR8 activity[62] as well as CpG oligonucleotides with TLR9 activity.[23,63,64] The monophosphoryl lipid A modification of bacterial LPS, a TLR4 agonist, has also been investigated as an adjuvant for *Leishmania* subunit vaccination.[65] We propose the use of topical TLR7/8 agonists as an adjuvant to whole-cell *Leishmania* vaccines because of their properties as activators of antigen-presenting cells, their propensity to redirect immune responses to a Th1 rather than a Th2 phenotype, and their potential modulating effects on regulatory T cells. These effects directly counteract many of the mechanisms that *Leishmania* species use to subvert the immune system in general (**Table 3**).

SUMMARY

Although the past challenges to develop effective vaccines against *Leishmania* parasites have been formidable, our exponentially increasing immunology knowledge base provides great hope for future developments. Although prior developments have led to increased understanding of infectious immunity in other systems, we proceed with caution to question dogmatic approaches to *Leishmania* immunity. What might seem like common sense immunology, if not scientifically tested, could skew scientific rationale. Vaccine strategies for leishmaniasis could suffer and end in the wrong direction. Exciting developments in other fields exemplify these notions, such as the role of memory T cells behaving like innate effector cells or B cells serving as antigen-presenting cells.[66] The importance of innate immunity and its role in the development of long-term protection against parasites cannot be overstated. The test is in the field, and we eagerly await the first successful vaccine against *Leishmania*.

REFERENCES

1. Kedzierski L. Leishmaniasis vaccine: where are we today? J Glob Infect Dis 2010;2(2):177–85.
2. Okwor I, Uzonna J. Vaccines and vaccination strategies against human cutaneous leishmaniasis. Hum Vaccin 2009;5(5):291–301.
3. Palatnik-de-Sousa CB. Vaccines for leishmaniasis in the fore coming 25 years. Vaccine 2008;26(14): 1709–24.
4. Reithinger R, Dujardin JC, Louzir H, et al. Cutaneous leishmaniasis. Lancet Infect Dis 2007;7(9):581–96.
5. Vanloubbeeck Y, Jones DE. The immunology of *Leishmania* infection and the implications for vaccine development. Ann N Y Acad Sci 2004; 1026:267–72.
6. Okwor I, Uzonna J. Persistent parasites and immunologic memory in cutaneous leishmaniasis: implications for vaccine designs and vaccination strategies. Immunol Res 2008;41(2):123–36.
7. Campos-Neto A. What about Th1/Th2 in cutaneous leishmaniasis vaccine discovery? Braz J Med Biol Res 2005;38(7):979–84.
8. Murray HW, Berman JD, Davies CR, et al. Advances in leishmaniasis. Lancet 2005;366(9496):1561–77.
9. David CV, Craft N. Cutaneous and mucocutaneous leishmaniasis. Dermatol Ther 2009;22(6):491–502.
10. Mitropoulos P, Konidas P, Durkin-Konidas M. New World cutaneous leishmaniasis: updated review of current and future diagnosis and treatment. J Am Acad Dermatol 2010;63(2):309–22.
11. Ezra N, Ochoa M, Craft N. Human immunodeficiency virus and leishmaniasis. J Global Infect Dis 2010;2:248–57.
12. Peters N, Sacks D. Immune privilege in sites of chronic infection: *Leishmania* and regulatory T cells. Immunol Rev 2006;213:159–79.

13. Sacks D, Noben-Trauth N. The immunology of susceptibility and resistance to *Leishmania major* in mice. Nat Rev Immunol 2002;2(11):845–58.

14. Belkaid Y, Piccirillo CA, Mendez S, et al. CD4+CD25+ regulatory T cells control *Leishmania major* persistence and immunity. Nature 2002; 420(6915):502–7.

15. Engwerda CR, Ato M, Kaye PM. Macrophages, pathology and parasite persistence in experimental visceral leishmaniasis. Trends Parasitol 2004;20(11):524–30.

16. Bekeredjian-Ding I, Jego G. Toll-like receptors—sentries in the B-cell response. Immunology 2009;128(3):311–23.

17. Brandonisio O, Spinelli R, Pepe M. Dendritic cells in *Leishmania* infection. Microbes Infect 2004; 6(15):1402–9.

18. Nylen S, Maurya R, Eidsmo L, et al. Splenic accumulation of IL-10 mRNA in T cells distinct from CD4+CD25+ (Foxp3) regulatory T cells in human visceral leishmaniasis. J Exp Med 2007;204(4): 805–17.

19. Gumy A, Louis JA, Launois P. The murine model of infection with *Leishmania major* and its importance for the deciphering of mechanisms underlying differences in Th cell differentiation in mice from different genetic backgrounds. Int J Parasitol 2004;34(4):433–44.

20. Reiner SL, Locksley RM. The regulation of immunity to *Leishmania major*. Annu Rev Immunol 1995;13: 151–77.

21. Wilson ME, Jeronimo SM, Pearson RD. Immunopathogenesis of infection with the visceralizing *Leishmania* species. Microb Pathog 2005;38(4):147–60.

22. Scott P. Development and regulation of cell-mediated immunity in experimental leishmaniasis. Immunol Res 2003;27(2-3):489–98.

23. Kebaier C, Uzonna JE, Beverley SM, et al. Immunization with persistent attenuated Delta lpg2 *Leishmania major* parasites requires adjuvant to provide protective immunity in C57BL/6 mice. Infect Immun 2006;74(1):777–80.

24. Perez LE, Chandrasekar B, Saldarriaga OA, et al. Reduced nitric oxide synthase 2 (NOS2) promoter activity in the Syrian hamster renders the animal functionally deficient in NOS2 activity and unable to control an intracellular pathogen. J Immunol 2006;176(9):5519–28.

25. Zaph C, Uzonna J, Beverley SM, et al. Central memory T cells mediate long-term immunity to *Leishmania major* in the absence of persistent parasites. Nat Med 2004;10(10):1104–10.

26. Scott P. Immunologic memory in cutaneous leishmaniasis. Cell Microbiol 2005;7(12):1707–13.

27. Akira S, Takeda K, Kaisho T. Toll-like receptors: critical proteins linking innate and acquired immunity. Nat Immunol 2001;2(8):675–80.

28. Dempsey PW, Vaidya SA, Cheng G. The art of war: Innate and adaptive immune responses. Cell Mol Life Sci 2003;60(12):2604–21.

29. Medzhitov R. Toll-like receptors and innate immunity. Nat Rev Immunol 2001;1(2):135–45.

30. Medzhitov R, Janeway C Jr. Innate immune recognition: mechanisms and pathways. Immunol Rev 2000;173:89–97.

31. Inohara N, Nunez G. NODs: intracellular proteins involved in inflammation and apoptosis. Nat Rev Immunol 2003;3(5):371–82.

32. Gomes IN, Palma LC, Campos GO, et al. The scavenger receptor MARCO is involved in *Leishmania major* infection by CBA/J macrophages. Parasite Immunol 2009;31(4):188–98.

33. Dabbagh K, Lewis DB. Toll-like receptors and T-helper-1/T-helper-2 responses. Curr Opin Infect Dis 2003;16(3):199–204.

34. Heil F, Hemmi H, Hochrein H, et al. Species-specific recognition of single-stranded RNA via toll-like receptor 7 and 8. Science 2004; 303(5663):1526–9.

35. Hemmi H, Kaisho T, Takeuchi O, et al. Small antiviral compounds activate immune cells via the TLR7 MyD88-dependent signaling pathway. Nat Immunol 2002;3(2):196–200.

36. de Veer MJ, Curtis JM, Baldwin TM, et al. MyD88 is essential for clearance of *Leishmania major*: possible role for lipophosphoglycan and Toll-like receptor 2 signaling. Eur J Immunol 2003;33(10): 2822–31.

37. Vaidya SA, Cheng G. Toll-like receptors and innate antiviral responses. Curr Opin Immunol 2003;15(4):402–7.

38. LaRosa DF, Gelman AE, Rahman AH, et al. CpG DNA inhibits CD4+CD25+ Treg suppression through direct MyD88-dependent costimulation of effector CD4+ T cells. Immunol Lett 2007;108(2):183–8.

39. Muraille E, De TC, Brait M, et al. Genetically resistant mice lacking MyD88-adapter protein display a high susceptibility to *Leishmania major* infection associated with a polarized Th2 response. J Immunol 2003;170(8):4237–41.

40. Tabbara KS. Progress towards a *Leishmania* vaccine. Saudi Med J 2006;27(7):942–50.

41. Tabbara KS, Peters NC, Afrin F, et al. Conditions influencing the efficacy of vaccination with live organisms against *Leishmania major* infection. Infect Immun 2005;73(8):4714–22.

42. Khamesipour A, Rafati S, Davoudi N, et al. Leishmaniasis vaccine candidates for development: a global overview. Indian J Med Res 2006;123(3): 423–38.

43. Noazin S, Khamesipour A, Moulton LH, et al. Efficacy of killed whole-parasite vaccines in the prevention of leishmaniasis: a meta-analysis. Vaccine 2009;27(35):4747–53.

44. Matzinger P. The danger model: a renewed sense of self. Science 2002;296(5566):301–5.

45. Montero Vega MT. A new era for innate immunity. Allergol Immunopathol (Madr) 2008;36(3):164–75.

46. Calvopina M, Barroso PA, Marco JD, et al. Efficacy of vaccination with a combination of Leishmania amastigote antigens and the lipid a-analogue ONO-4007 for immunoprophylaxis and immunotherapy against Leishmania amazonensis infection in a murine model of new world cutaneous leishmaniasis. Vaccine 2006;24(27–28):5645–52.

47. Dondji B, Perez-Jimenez E, Goldsmith-Pestana K, et al. Heterologous prime-boost vaccination with the LACK antigen protects against murine visceral leishmaniasis. Infect Immun 2005;73(8):5286–9.

48. Garg R, Dube A. Animal models for vaccine studies for visceral leishmaniasis. Indian J Med Res 2006;123(3):439–54.

49. Kedzierski L, Zhu Y, Handman E. Leishmania vaccines: progress and problems. Parasitology 2006;133(Suppl):S87–112.

50. Sidky YA, Borden EC, Weeks CE, et al. Inhibition of murine tumor growth by an interferon-inducing imidazoquinolinamine. Cancer Res 1992;52(13):3528–33.

51. Bernstein DI, Harrison CJ. Effects of the immunomodulating agent R837 on acute and latent herpes simplex virus type 2 infections. Antimicrob Agents Chemother 1989;33(9):1511–5.

52. Gorden KB, Gorski KS, Gibson SJ, et al. Synthetic TLR agonists reveal functional differences between human TLR7 and TLR8. J Immunol 2005;174(3):1259–68.

53. Testerman TL, Gerster JF, Imbertson LM, et al. Cytokine induction by the immunomodulators imiquimod and S-27609. J Leukoc Biol 1995;58(3):365–72.

54. Gibson SJ, Imbertson LM, Wagner TL, et al. Cellular requirements for cytokine production in response to the immunomodulators imiquimod and S-27609. J Interferon Cytokine Res 1995;15(6):537–45.

55. Megyeri K, Au WC, Rosztoczy I, et al. Stimulation of interferon and cytokine gene expression by imiquimod and stimulation by Sendai virus utilize similar signal transduction pathways. Mol Cell Biol 1995;15(4):2207–18.

56. Nair S, McLaughlin C, Weizer A, et al. Injection of immature dendritic cells into adjuvant-treated skin obviates the need for ex vivo maturation. J Immunol 2003;171(11):6275–82.

57. Doxsee CL, Riter TR, Reiter MJ, et al. The immune response modifier and Toll-like receptor 7 agonist S-27609 selectively induces IL-12 and TNF-alpha production in CD11c+CD11b+CD8- dendritic cells. J Immunol 2003;171(3):1156–63.

58. Otero M, Calarota SA, Felber B, et al. Resiquimod is a modest adjuvant for HIV-1 gag-based genetic immunization in a mouse model. Vaccine 2004;22(13-14):1782–90.

59. Yi H, Zhen Y, Jiang L, et al. The phenotypic characterization of naturally occurring regulatory CD4+CD25+ T cells. Cell Mol Immunol 2006;3(3):189–95.

60. Arevalo I, Ward B, Miller R, et al. Successful treatment of drug-resistant cutaneous leishmaniasis in humans by use of imiquimod, an immunomodulator. Clin Infect Dis 2001;33(11):1847–51.

61. Buates S, Matlashewski G. Treatment of experimental leishmaniasis with the immunomodulators imiquimod and S-28463: Efficacy and mode of action. J Infect Dis 1999;179:1485–94.

62. Zhang WW, Matlashewski G. Immunization with a Toll-like receptor 7 and/or 8 agonist vaccine adjuvant increases protective immunity against Leishmania major in BALB/c mice. Infect Immun 2008;76(8):3777–83.

63. Wu W, Weigand L, Belkaid Y, et al. Immunomodulatory effects associated with a live vaccine against Leishmania major containing CpG oligodeoxynucleotides. Eur J Immunol 2006;36(12):3238–47.

64. Flynn B, Wang V, Sacks DL, et al. Prevention and treatment of cutaneous leishmaniasis in primates by using synthetic type D/A oligodeoxynucleotides expressing CpG motifs. Infect Immun 2005;73(8):4948–54.

65. Coler RN, Reed SG. Second-generation vaccines against leishmaniasis. Trends Parasitol 2005;21(5):244–9.

66. Ronet C, Voigt H, Himmelrich H, et al. Leishmania major-specific B cells are necessary for Th2 cell development and susceptibility to L. major LV39 in BALB/c mice. J Immunol 2008;180(7):4825–35.

67. Bomfim G, Andrade BB, Santos S, et al. Cellular analysis of cutaneous leishmaniasis lymphadenopathy: insights into the early phases of human disease. Am J Trop Med Hyg 2007;77(5):854–9.

68. Peters NC, Egen JG, Secundino N, et al. In vivo imaging reveals an essential role for neutrophils in leishmaniasis transmitted by sand flies. Science 2008;321(5891):970–4.

69. Guimaraes-Costa AB, Nascimento MT, Froment GS, et al. Leishmania amazonensis promastigotes induce and are killed by neutrophil extracellular traps. Proc Natl Acad Sci U S A 2009;106(16):6748–53.

70. Peters NC, Sacks DL. The impact of vector-mediated neutrophil recruitment on cutaneous leishmaniasis. Cell Microbiol 2009;11(9):1290–6.

71. Charmoy M, Megnekou R, Allenbach C, et al. Leishmania major induces distinct neutrophil phenotypes in mice that are resistant or susceptible to infection. J Leukoc Biol 2007;82(2):288–99.

72. Novais FO, Santiago RC, Bafica A, et al. Neutrophils and macrophages cooperate in host

resistance against *Leishmania braziliensis* infection. J Immunol 2009;183(12):8088–98.

73. Peters NC, Kimblin N, Secundino N, et al. Vector transmission of *Leishmania* abrogates vaccine-induced protective immunity. PLoS Pathog 2009; 5(6):e1000484.

74. Flandin JF, Chano F, Descoteaux A. RNA interference reveals a role for TLR2 and TLR3 in the recognition of *Leishmania donovani* promastigotes by interferon-gamma-primed macrophages. Eur J Immunol 2006;36(2):411–20.

75. Gomez MA, Contreras I, Halle M, et al. *Leishmania* GP63 alters host signaling through cleavage-activated protein tyrosine phosphatases. Sci Signal 2009;2(90):ra58.

76. Arendse B, Van Snick J, Brombacher F. IL-9 is a susceptibility factor in *Leishmania major* infection by promoting detrimental Th2/type 2 responses. J Immunol 2005;174(4):2205–11.

77. Wanasen N, Soong L. ʟ-Arginine metabolism and its impact on host immunity against *Leishmania* infection. Immunol Res 2008;41(1):15–25.

78. Bowdle A, Kharasch E, Schwid H. Pressure waveform monitoring during central venous catheterization. Anesth Analg 2009;109(6):2030–1; author reply 2031.

79. Soong L. Modulation of dendritic cell function by *Leishmania* parasites. J Immunol 2008;180(7): 4355–60.

80. Liese J, Schleicher U, Bogdan C. The innate immune response against *Leishmania* parasites. Immunobiology 2008;213(3-4):377–87.

81. Laabs EM, Wu W, Mendez S. Vaccination with live *Leishmania major* and CpG DNA promotes interleukin-2 production by dermal dendritic cells and NK cell activation. Clin Vaccine Immunol 2009;16(11):1601–6.

82. Vargas-Inchaustegui DA, Tai W, Xin L, et al. Distinct roles for MyD88 and Toll-like receptor 2 during *Leishmania braziliensis* infection in mice. Infect Immun 2009;77(7):2948–56.

83. Ng LG, Hsu A, Mandell MA, et al. Migratory dermal dendritic cells act as rapid sensors of protozoan parasites. PLoS Pathog 2008;4(11):e1000222.

84. Liu D, Kebaier C, Pakpour N, et al. *Leishmania major* phosphoglycans influence the host early immune response by modulating dendritic cell functions. Infect Immun 2009;77(8):3272–83.

85. Ramirez-Pineda JR, Frohlich A, Berberich C, et al. Dendritic cells (DC) activated by CpG DNA ex vivo are potent inducers of host resistance to an intracellular pathogen that is independent of IL-12 derived from the immunizing DC. J Immunol 2004;172(10):6281–9.

86. Wiethe C, Debus A, Mohrs M, et al. Dendritic cell differentiation state and their interaction with NKT cells determine Th1/Th2 differentiation in the murine model of *Leishmania major* infection. J Immunol 2008;180(7):4371–81.

87. De Trez C, Magez S, Akira S, et al. iNOS-producing inflammatory dendritic cells constitute the major infected cell type during the chronic *Leishmania major* infection phase of C57BL/6 resistant mice. PLoS Pathog 2009;5(6):e1000494.

88. Becker I, Salaiza N, Aguirre M, et al. *Leishmania* lipophosphoglycan (LPG) activates NK cells through toll-like receptor-2. Mol Biochem Parasitol 2003;130(2):65–74.

89. Nylen S, Maasho K, Soderstrom K, et al. Live *Leishmania* promastigotes can directly activate primary human natural killer cells to produce interferon-gamma. Clin Exp Immunol 2003;131(3):457–67.

90. Nylen S, Maasho K, McMahon-Pratt D, et al. Leishmanial amastigote antigen P-2 induces major histocompatibility complex class II-dependent natural killer-cell reactivity in cells from healthy donors. Scand J Immunol 2004;59(3):294–304.

91. Manna PP, Chakrabarti G, Bandyopadhyay S. Innate immune defense in visceral leishmaniasis: cytokine mediated protective role by allogeneic effector cell. Vaccine 2010;28(3):803–10.

92. Maurer M, Lopez Kostka S, Siebenhaar F, et al. Skin mast cells control T cell-dependent host defense in *Leishmania major* infections. FASEB J 2006;20(14):2460–7.

93. Villasenor-Cardoso MI, Salaiza N, Delgado J, et al. Mast cells are activated by *Leishmania mexicana* LPG and regulate the disease outcome depending on the genetic background of the host. Parasite Immunol 2008. [Epub ahead of print].

94. Romao PR, Da Costa Santiago H, Ramos CD, et al. Mast cell degranulation contributes to susceptibility to *Leishmania major.* Parasite Immunol 2009; 31(3):140–6.

95. Revaz-Breton M, Ronet C, Ives A, et al. The MyD88 protein 88 pathway is differently involved in immune responses induced by distinct substrains of *Leishmania major.* Eur J Immunol 2010;40(6):1697–707.

96. Uzonna JE, Spath GF, Beverley SM, et al. Vaccination with phosphoglycan-deficient *Leishmania major* protects highly susceptible mice from virulent challenge without inducing a strong Th1 response. J Immunol 2004;172(6):3793–7.

97. Kavoosi G, Ardestani SK, Kariminia A, et al. *Leishmania major* lipophosphoglycan: discrepancy in Toll-like receptor signaling. Exp Parasitol 2010; 124(2):214–8.

98. Guerra CS, Macedo Silva RM, Carvalho LO, et al. Histopathological analysis of initial cellular response in TLR-2 deficient mice experimentally infected by *Leishmania (L) amazonensis.* Int J Exp Pathol 2010. [Epub ahead of print].

99. Kavoosi G, Ardestani SK, Kariminia A. The involvement of TLR2 in cytokine and reactive oxygen

species (ROS) production by PBMCs in response to *Leishmania major* phosphoglycans (PGs). Parasitology 2009;136(10):1193–9.

100. Kropf P, Freudenberg MA, Modolell M, et al. Toll-like receptor 4 contributes to efficient control of infection with the protozoan parasite *Leishmania major*. Infect Immun 2004;72(4):1920–8.

101. Zimmermann S, Dalpke A, Heeg K. CpG oligonucleotides as adjuvant in therapeutic vaccines against parasitic infections. Int J Med Microbiol 2008;298(1–2):39–44.

102. Kropf P, Fuentes JM, Fahnrich E, et al. Arginase and polyamine synthesis are key factors in the regulation of experimental leishmaniasis in vivo. FASEB J 2005;19(8):1000–2.

103. Rocha FJ, Schleicher U, Mattner J, et al. Cytokines, signaling pathways, and effector molecules required for the control of *Leishmania (Viannia) braziliensis* in mice. Infect Immun 2007;75(8):3823–32.

104. Moreno I, Dominguez M, Cabanes D, et al. Kinetic analysis of ex vivo human blood infection by *Leishmania*. PLoS Negl Trop Dis 2010;4(7):e743.

105. Kedzierski L, Montgomery J, Bullen D, et al. A leucine-rich repeat motif of *Leishmania* parasite surface antigen 2 binds to macrophages through the complement receptor 3. J Immunol 2004; 172(8):4902–6.

106. Mangsbo SM, Sanchez J, Anger K, et al. Complement activation by CpG in a human whole blood loop system: mechanisms and immunomodulatory effects. J Immunol 2009;183(10):6724–32.

107. McGwire BS, Kulkarni MM. Interactions of antimicrobial peptides with *Leishmania* and trypanosomes and their functional role in host parasitism. Exp Parasitol 2010;126(3):397–405.

108. Teixeira CR, Teixeira MJ, Gomes RB, et al. Saliva from *Lutzomyia longipalpis* induces CC chemokine ligand 2/monocyte chemoattractant protein-1 expression and macrophage recruitment. J Immunol 2005; 175(12):8346–53.

109. Gomes R, Teixeira C, Teixeira MJ, et al. Immunity to a salivary protein of a sand fly vector protects against the fatal outcome of visceral leishmaniasis in a hamster model. Proc Natl Acad Sci U S A 2008;105(22):7845–50.

110. Oliveira F, Lawyer PG, Kamhawi S, et al. Immunity to distinct sand fly salivary proteins primes the anti-*Leishmania* immune response towards protection or exacerbation of disease. PLoS Negl Trop Dis 2008;2(4):e226.

Female Genital Mutilation: What Every American Dermatologist Needs to Know

Amish J. Dave, MD[a],*, Aisha Sethi, MD[b],
Aldo Morrone, MD, PhD[c]

KEYWORDS

- Female genital mutilation • Female circumcision
- International dermatology • Tropical dermatology
- Human rights

Female genital mutilation (FGM) is a condition with which dermatologists should be familiarized, as it likely will be seen with rising frequency in the American dermatologist's clinic. With increased immigration of individuals from regions where the practice is endemic to the United States and other industrialized nations, FGM has gained growing attention.[1] FGM was formally defined by the World Health Organization (WHO), United Nations Population Fund (UNFPA), and the United Nations Children's Fund (UNICEF) as that which

> "comprises all procedures involving partial or total removal of the external female genitalia or other injury to the female genital organs whether for cultural or other non-therapeutic reasons[2]"

Estimates of the prevalence of the practice vary on a regional basis, with WHO estimating in 1998 that 137 million women underwent the procedure, and a further two million girls are at risk each year.[3] In the United States, an estimated 168,000 women in 1990 were believed to either have undergone or to be at risk of FGM (**Fig. 1**).[4]

While the practice of altering a woman or girl's genitalia has been alternatively termed circumcision or ritual female genital surgery among other names, the term mutilation may best convey the sheer impact of the procedure on both a psychological and physical sense.[5] FGM is known to be associated with innumerable changes in a female's life, from decreased fertility[6] to increased risk of dermatologic complications[1] to potentially elevated risk of human immunodeficiency virus (HIV) contraction.[7,8] Dermatologists seeking to reduce the incidence of FGM must be cognizant of the risks to victims arising from the practice, but also understand that FGM is a form of child and female abuse that is both medically dangerous and socially unacceptable in that it ultimately victimizes women.[4]

This article aims to (1) explain the widely used WHO classification system for FGM, (2) discuss the prevalence of FGM in the United States, (3) provide a review on dermatologic complications of the procedure, and (4) offer suggestions to dermatologists working with women who have been victims of FGM.

The authors have nothing to disclose.
[a] Department of Medicine, Stanford University School of Medicine, 300 Pasteur Drive, Grant S101, Stanford, CA 94305-5109, USA
[b] Section of Dermatology, Department of Medicine, University of Chicago Medical Center, 5841 South Maryland Avenue MC 5067, Chicago, IL 60637, USA
[c] National institute for Health, Migration and Poverty, Via di San Gallicano 25/a, 00153 Roma, Italy
* Corresponding author.
E-mail address: AJDave6@uchicago.edu

Dermatol Clin 29 (2011) 103–109
doi:10.1016/j.det.2010.09.002
0733-8635/11/$ — see front matter © 2011 Elsevier Inc. All rights reserved.

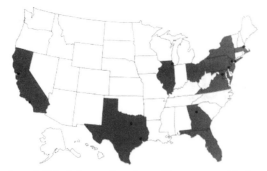

Fig. 1. US states and metropolitan areas with the largest estimated numbers of women and girls with or at risk for female genital mutilation/female circumcision (FGM/FC), 1990. The Centers for Disease Control and Prevention (CDC) have developed a statistical model to estimate the number of girls and women with or at risk for FGM/FC living in the United States. Some 168,000 girls or women were estimated using 1990 census data to have received or to be at risk for these procedures. States with large African immigrant populations were found to have the greatest numbers of girls and women with or potentially at risk for FGM/FC. An estimated 45% of the women and 44% of the girls younger than age 18 estimated to have or be at risk for FGM/FC lived in 11 metropolitan areas. (*Data from* Jones WK, Smith J, Kieke B Jr, et al. Female genital mutilation: female circumcision; who is at risk in the US? Public Health Rep 1997;112:368.)

CLASSIFICATION

Currently, the WHO, UNFPA, and UNICEF have classified FGM into four types (**Fig. 2**)[9]:

> Type 1. Clitoridectomy: partial or total removal of the clitoris, with or without removal of the prepuce.

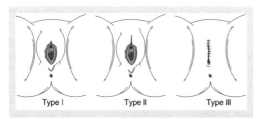

Fig. 2. World Health Organization classification of female genital cutting. Type I, also known as clitoridectomy or sunna, involves removing part or all of the clitoris and/or the prepuce. Type II, also known as excision, involves removing part or all of the clitoris and labia minora, with or without excision of the labia majora. Type III, the most severe form, is also called infibulation or pharaonic. It entails removing part or all of the external genitalia and narrowing the vaginal orifice by reapproximating the labia minora and/or labia majora. (*From* Nour NM. Female genital cutting: clinical and cultural guidelines. Obstet Gynecol Surv 2004;59:272–9; with permission.)

Type 2. Excision: partial or total removal of the clitoris and labia minora, with or without excision of the labia majora.

Type 3. Infibulation: narrowing of the vaginal opening through creation of a covering seal. The seal is formed by cutting and then moving the inner (and sometimes the outer) labia. Infibulation may be performed with or without clitoral excision. This practice is the most severe form of FGM. Women must have their legs bound for a period of 1 to 4 weeks following the procedure to allow for healing of tissues and fusion of the labia majora. Deinfibulation, or the widening of the vaginal opening (typically before childbirth), is either performed by the husband during intercourse or by a physician or FGM practitioner. Following childbirth, a woman may have a reinfibulation procedure, whereby her vaginal opening is once again narrowed.[10]

Type 4. All other harmful procedures to the female genitalia for any nontherapeutic purpose, including pricking, piercing, incising, scraping, and cauterizing of the genital area.

While the joint classification scheme aims to aid researchers and health care professionals in standardizing their descriptions of multiple operations,[1,11] practitioners of FGM rarely refer to the procedures they perform by WHO type. With often only a cursory knowledge of the procedures themselves, victims often underestimate the extent of their genital alterations.[12] FGM is frequently conducted by elderly women who are assigned to the practice by community members or by midwives. The procedure tends to last less than 20 minutes and involves instruments such as special knives, scissors, scalpels, pieces of glass, or razor blades that rarely are sanitized adequately and are reused frequently.[1]

EPIDEMIOLOGY AND PREVALENCE

Genital modification has been practiced by various peoples in Africa, Southeast Asia, South Asia, and the Middle East for centuries.[1] While the practice is widespread, Africa is the hotbed of FGM and the place where both the mildest and most brutal forms are conducted.[13] While many types of FGM are conducted in every African country, Nour[6] (2008) noted that type 1 FGM is practiced primarily in Ethiopia, Eritrea, and Kenya; type 2 is practiced in parts of West Africa, including Benin, Sierra Leone, Gambia, and Guinea; and type 3 is practiced in Somalia, northern Sudan, and Djibouti

(**Fig. 3**). Information on current practice of genital mutilation in Africa arises from some large nation-wide surveys and numerous smaller studies. While each study has its individual strengths and flaws, these surveys are all too often complicated by small sample sizes, nonrepresentative groups, irregularities in participant selection, and haphazard data collection.[1]

Surveys attempting to estimate the number of women who have experienced FGM or are at risk of FGM in the industrialized world suffer from design and selection problems similar to those in the third world. In 1996, the US Congress directed the US Department of Health and Human Services to produce an estimate of the number of girls and women who had undergone FGM or are at risk. Based on 1990 census data (which used a 5% sample of the estimated entire US population) and available prevalence estimates in 27 African countries, Jones and colleagues[4] (1997) estimated that 168,000 out of 271,000 African immigrants in the United States were at risk of FGM. Their study relied on the assumption that African immigrants would perform FGM at rates similar to individuals in their homelands regardless of when the emigration occurred or where in the United States the immigrants settled. The researchers found that 77.1% of at-risk women lived in 12 states (California, Florida, Georgia, Illinois, Maryland, Massachusetts, New Jersey, New York, Ohio, Texas, and Virginia) and the District of Columbia, while 45% of endangered women lived in 11 metropolitan cities. These cities include New York City, Washington, DC,

Los-Angeles-Long Beach, Houston, Chicago, Philadelphia (including suburban New Jersey), Atlanta, Oakland, California, Newark, New Jersey, Dallas, and Boston (including suburban New Hampshire) (see **Fig. 1**).

While the study has allowed a number to be attached to the idea of at-risk women, the authors acknowledged that a more precise determination of risk was complicated by the small number of African immigrants questioned in the US Census and the fact that many immigrants gave no country of origin in the census other than Africa. For individuals who gave only a region of origin (43% of the sample), weighted regional prevalence of FGM was used. Furthermore, the estimate did not take into account the age of emigration, the age at which FGM is practiced in the native culture, the length of residence and degree of acculturation in the United States, or whether immigrants differed in education, beliefs, or family history of FGM from individuals in their homelands.[4] Although the United States may well have the most at-risk women in the industrialized world, European nations also have been noting large numbers of women who have undergone or are at risk of FGM. Upwards of 20,000 girls in the United Kingdom have been estimated to be endangered, while a 1989 report in France suggested that 20,000 women and 12,500 girls either had suffered or would suffer FGM in that country.[13–15] A recent Swiss review suggested that the alpine nation might be home to around 6000 girls and women with FGM.[16] These

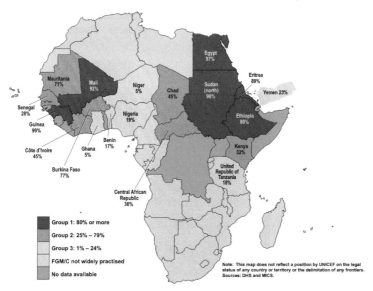

Fig. 3. Female genital cutting prevalence among women aged 15–49 years. (*Adapted from* Demographic and health surveys and multiple indicator cluster surveys. Female genital mutilation/cutting: a statistical exploration. New York: UNICEF; 2005:4.)

estimates lend further credibility to the idea that FGM can no longer be thought of as a condition of underdeveloped nations, but, rather, that it must be addressed as a genuine concern in the industrialized world.

DERMATOLOGIC COMPLICATIONS OF FGM

There is no shortage of medical literature highlighting complications arising from various forms of FGM. Morrone and colleagues[1] (2002) wrote a summary of FGM complications. In addition to numerous psychiatric sequelae, FGM has multiple short-term complications (ie, death, shock, tetanus, and failure of wound healing), obstetric and gynecologic complications (ie, infertility, potentially enhanced risk of HIV and sexually transmitted diseases (STDs), complications in delivery, and risk of intrapartum hemorrhage), and urological problems (ie, vesicovaginal fistulae, injury to the urethra, and difficulty in passing urine). Furthermore, there is active debate on whether FGM increases transmission of HIV and other STDs.[7,8,17]

The dermatologic findings of FGM have been extensively reported in case reports and include keloids, epidermoid cysts, clitoral neuromas, and scarification (**Fig. 4**). Deep tissue cuts may exacerbate keloids and hypertrophic scars while increasing the risk of abscesses. In addition, inflammation secondary to both postmutilation infections and poor urinary drainage has been suggested to play a role in particularly severe keloid formation in FGM patients.[1] Women may delay treatment of keloids in the genital region for years because of embarrassment or fear of surgical options. Certainly, although never formally studied, particularly large keloids can only contribute to the obstetric complications associated with genital mutilation.

The most common dermatologic complication of FGM, however, has been the development of epidermal inclusion cysts (EICs) in the genital area, with multiple case reports in the medical literature of women developing cysts decades after being cut.[18–22] One 1-year study of women admitted to a hospital in northwestern Somalia with circumcision complications noted EICs in 55% (65 of 118) of patients.[20] Another survey by the same authors in Mogadishu, Somalia, noted that 12.4% (36 of 290 patients) developed EICs after infibulations.[23] Although treatment of such cysts is often simple surgical excision with removal of the intact cyst or, more recently, by carbon dioxide laser surgery,[24] women may experience years of pelvic or abdominal pain, dyspareunia, pruritus, and discharge associated with EICs.[19,20,23] Larger cysts may pose complications to vaginal delivery and might require prenatal excision.[24]

In addition to cyst development, pelvic pain in FGM victims also may be associated with amputation neuromas of the clitoris.[25] Such neuromas may arise secondary to clitoral nerve entrapment in haphazardly placed stitches by the FGM practitioner or due to development of scar tissue that increases pressure on the nerve. Women with amputation neuromas may suffer from decades of dyspareunia or pain at rest and require careful surgical excision of the trapped nerve.[1]

FGM has been said to lead to increased risk of acquiring sexually transmitted infections (STIs) and their complications, such as pelvic inflammatory diseases (PID), but still little is

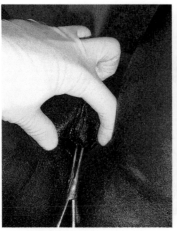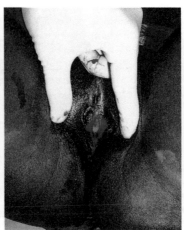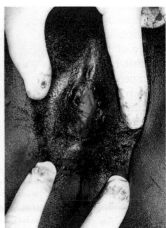

Fig. 4. Deinfibulation to reveal clitoridectomy and excision of the labia as seen in type III female genital mutilation. (*Courtesy of* Dr Hassan Azadeh and David Ellis, The University of Gambia Medical School, 2010; with permission.)

known about the relation of this practice and STIs. In spite of the known complications and the potential for HIV transmission through FGM, there are very limited studies reviewing this practice currently and presenting perspective on the probability of FGM leading to HIV transmission. Biologically, any sexually related viral or bacterial pathogen has increased propensity for transmission, given trauma or pre-existing laceration to the vaginal epithelium. FGM increases the risk of vaginal epithelial damage and consequently increases the probability of HIV transmission.[1] HIV transmission from FGM practice is enhanced through shared instruments and blood products during the practice of genital cutting as well as damage to the vaginal epithelium associated with the trauma, inflammation, and complications. Other modes of HIV transmission, as well as other HIV risk factors, may occur in association with this practice, making it difficult to ascertain whether FGM is the sole predisposing risk factor, as well as a contributing variable to the cumulative incidence of HIV in sub-Saharan Africa.[1]

LEGAL AND SOCIAL ISSUES SURROUNDING FGM PRACTICE

Unless deemed necessary by health care professionals to protect a woman's health, the practice of FGM is a federal criminal offense in the United States. In 1997, the US Congress passed a federal appropriations bill (P.L. 104–208) that included a provision stating that any individual who conducts FGM on a woman under the age of 18 would be either imprisoned not more than 5 years or fined or both. The US Congress reaffirmed its commitment to ending FGM when it enacted a provision criminalizing the practice as part of the Illegal Immigration Reform and Immigrant Responsibility Act of 2006 for all women under the age of 18. Currently, however, there are no laws that refer to acceptable treatment options for women who have undergone FGM, including under what circumstances reinfibulation is acceptable practice.[26]

As of 2004, 16 states had passed legislation relating to FGM. In general, these statewide statutes address FGM in a manner similar to that of federal law by prohibiting its practice and instituting criminal sanctions. Out of these 16 states, three states (Minnesota, Rhode Island, and Tennessee) prohibit the practice of FGM on adult women as well as on all girls under the age of 18.[26] Particularly stringent is Illinois' criminal code amendment that went into effect on Jan. 1, 1998. The law states that "whoever knowingly circumcises, excises, or infibulates, in whole or in part, the labia majora, labia minora, or clitoris of another commits the offense of female genital mutilation." FGM is a class X felony, punishable by not less than 6 years or more than 30 years imprisonment. The statute prohibits the performance of FGM on both minors and adults.[26] While these steps are to be commended, one of the challenges to lowering the incidence of FGM will be to pair the passage of laws against the practice with more consistent law enforcement and targeted education campaigns in communities where FGM is widely practiced. Although many state laws may include special provisions instructing state officials to develop education programs for physicians and communities where FGM is common, these provisions are all too often nonuniform, unfunded, and uncoordinated.

SUMMARY

Several reasons have been given for why genital mutilation is still widely performed, challenging the idea that male dominance or any one single cause underlies FGM.[27] Parents who seek FGM usually love their daughters and wish for the procedure because they believe that it is in their best interest. Parents may believe that FGM will increase their daughter's fertility or ability to please her spouse sexually, make her more marriageable and devout, ensure her virginity, or be a sign of beauty and good hygiene.[6,28] Others have noted traditional beliefs that the clitoris is toxic and might harm infants during the birthing process, the idea that the clitoris must be cut to prevent it from growing toward the ground, and the thought that clitoridectomies enhance survival and reputation.[6]

Dermatologists in the United States should expect to see a growing number of patients having undergone FGM who may present with complications such as keloids, epidermoid cysts, clitoral neuromas, and abscess formation. As Jaeger and colleagues[28] (2009) have noted, one challenge for dermatologists and other health care professionals will be to maintain a neutral, respectful, and unemotional attitude when approaching the issue of FGM. Individuals from cultures where FGM is endemic are aware that Westerners tend to view genital cutting with abhorrence and are likely to be wary of discussing the topic with dermatologists. Although FGM should never be condoned, a discussion on the topic in the clinic should begin with a respectful introduction, focusing on ascertaining family members' thoughts on FGM and providing detailed information on medical and legal complications. Support structures for the family and social resources should be determined and arguments for performing FGM gently, but firmly debunked.[1]

The eradication of genital mutilation will ultimately require the use of multiple societal resources, all of which must play a delicate role in persuading parents not to support FGM while preventing the stigmatization and isolation of immigrants concerned about losing their values in alien countries. Ultimately, it is important to recognize that, although great harm arises from all forms of FGM, the parents who support the practice love their daughters.[2] As Gruenbaum[27] (2005) has so eloquently noted, "Regardless of the emotional or moral response people feel, those who are committed to abolition will be most effective if the change efforts are sophisticated, culturally informed, and socially contextualized."[3] In fighting to end FGM, emphasizing that love of one's daughter also means taking greater responsibility for her well-being and health may be the best and most universal argument in the arsenal against an ancient and devastating practice.

ACKNOWLEDGMENT

Nida Shakir, BA, was instrumental in researching legal and social issues surrounding the practice of FGM in the United States.

REFERENCES

1. Morrone A, Hercogova J, Lotti T. Stop female genital mutilation: appeal to the international dermatologic community. Int J Dermatol 2002;41(5):253–63.
2. World Health Organization. Female genital mutilation: a joint WHO/UNICEF/UNFPA statement. Geneva (Switzerland): World Health Organization; 1997. p. 1–6.
3. World Health Organization. Female genital mutilation: an overview. Geneva (Switzerland): World Health Organization; 1998. p. 1–6.
4. Jones WK, Smith J, Kieke B Jr, Wilcox L. Female genital mutilation: female circumcision; who is at risk in the US? Public Health Rep 1997;112:368.
5. Almroth L, Elmusharaf S, El Hadi N, et al. Primary infertility after genital mutilation in girlhood in Sudan: a case–control study. Lancet 2005;366(9483):385–91.
6. Nour NM. Female genital cutting: a persisting practice. Rev Obstet Gynecol 2008;1(3):135–9.
7. Klouman E, Manongi R, Klepp KI. Self-reported and observed female genital cutting in rural Tanzania: associated demographic factors, HIV, and sexually transmitted infections. Trop Med Int Health 2005; 10(1):105–15.
8. Rushwan H. Female genital mutilation (FGM) management during pregnancy, childbirth, and the postpartum period. Int J Gynaecol Obstet 2000; 70(1):99–104.
9. World Health Organization. Female genital mutilation. Available at: http://www.who.int/mediacentre/factsheets/fs241/en/index.html. Accessed November 15, 2009.
10. Arbesman M, Kahler L, Buck GM. Assessment of the impact of female circumcision on the gynecological, genitourinary and obstetrical health problems of women from Somalia: literature review and case series. Women Health 1993;20(3):27–42.
11. Toubia N. Female genital mutilation: a call for global action. 2nd edition. New York: RAIMB8; 1995.
12. Elmusharaf S, Elhadi N, Almroth L. Reliability of self reported form of female genital mutilation and WHO classification: cross-sectional study. BMJ 2006; 333(7559):124.
13. Eke N, Nkanginieme KE. Female genital mutilation: a global bug that should not cross the millennium bridge. World J Surg 1999;23(10):1082–7.
14. Robson A. Torture not culture. Amnesty Int Br Sec J 1993;8:9.
15. Gallard C. Female genital mutilation in France. BMJ 1995;310:1592.
16. Thierfelder C, Tanner M, Bodiang CM. Female genital mutilation in the context of migration: experience of African women with the Swiss health care system. Eur J Public Health 2005; 15(1):86–90.
17. Kun KE. Female genital mutilation: the potential for increased risk of HIV infection. Int J Gynaecol Obstet 1997;59:153–5.
18. Ofodile FA, Oluwasanmi JO. Postcircumcision epidermoid inclusion cysts of the clitoris. Plast Reconstr Surg 1979;63(4):485–6.
19. Hanly MG, Ojeda VJ. Epidermal inclusion cysts of the clitoris as a complication of female circumcision and pharaonic infibulation. Cent Afr J Med 1995; 41(1):22–4.
20. Kroll GL, Miller L. Vulvar epithelial inclusion cyst as a late complication of childhood female traditional genital surgery. Am J Obstet Gynecol 2000;183(2): 509–10.
21. Moreira PM, Moreira IV, Faye EH, et al. Three cases of epidermal cyst of vulva following female genital mutilation. Gynecol Obstet Fertil 2002;30: 958–60.
22. Al-Maghrabi J, Kanaan H, Bondagji N. Postcircumcision epidermoid inclusion cyst of the vulva containing multiple stones. Int J Gynaecol Obstet 2005; 90(2):155–6.
23. Rouzi AA, Sindi O, Radhan B, et al. Epidermal clitoral inclusion cyst after type I female genital mutilation. Am J Obstet Gynecol 2001;185(3): 569–71.
24. Penna C, Fallani MG, Fambrini M, et al. Type III female genital mutilation: clinical implications and

treatment by carbon dioxide laser surgery. Am J Obstet Gynecol 2002;187(6):1550–4.

25. Fernández-Aguilar S, Noël JC. Neuroma of the clitoris after female genital cutting. Obstet Gynecol 2003;101(5):1053–4.

26. Legislation on female genital mutilation in the United States. Center for Reproductive Rights. Available at: http://reproductiverights.org/en/document/female-genital-mutilation-fgm-legal-prohibitions-worldwide. Accessed December 2, 2009.

27. Gruenbaum E. Sociocultural dynamics of female genital cutting: research findings, gaps, and directions. Cult Health Sex 2005;7(5):429–41.

28. Jaeger F, Caflisch M, Hohlfeld P. Female genital mutilation and its prevention: a challenge for paediatricians. Eur J Pediatr 2009;168(1):27–33.

Widespread Use of Toxic Skin Lightening Compounds: Medical and Psychosocial Aspects

Barry Ladizinski, MD[a], Nisha Mistry, MD[b], Roopal V. Kundu, MD[c],*

KEYWORDS

- Skin lightening • Skin bleaching
- Skin whitening • Hydroquinone
- Exogenous ochronosis • Mercury poisoning
- Topical corticosteroids • Hyperpigmentation

Disorders of hyperpigmentation and skin lightening treatments have a significant impact on the dermatologic, physiologic, psychologic, economic, social, and cultural aspects of life. Skin lightening compounds or bleaching agents are chemicals used to achieve a lighter skin tone or whiten skin. These compounds are commonly used by individuals with hyperpigmentation disorders, such as melasma and postinflammatory hyperpigmentation (PIH), or those that desire lighter skin for cosmetic reasons. The most commonly used skin lightening products contain hydroquinone, topical corticosteroids (TCs), or mercury. Despite their apparent effectiveness, numerous cutaneous and systemic complications have been associated with these agents (Table 1), resulting in more stringent regulations regarding the preparation and distribution of skin lightening products. In addition to the medical implications and patient safety concerns, the psychosocial aspects of hyperpigmentation disorders are important to consider, particularly their impact on quality of life, to further elucidate the motivations for skin bleaching.

MEDICAL USE OF TOPICAL SKIN LIGHTENING COMPOUNDS

Hydroquinone

The most commonly used over-the-counter (OTC) and prescription skin lightening preparation is a ubiquitous phenol compound known as hydroquinone or 1,4-dihydroxybenzene.[1] Topical application of hydroquinone competitively inhibits melanogenesis through suppression of tyrosinase[2] and subsequent release of semiquinone free radicals, which are toxic to melanosomes.[3] In rat and human skin in vitro studies, hydroquinone has been shown to penetrate the epidermis and continue into the dermis, subcutaneous tissue, and circulation.[4]

Hydroquinone's ability to lighten skin was first reported by Oettel in 1936,[5] when hydroquinone ingestion caused pigmentation changes in

Disclosures: The authors have nothing to disclose; Funding sources: none.
[a] Department of Internal Medicine, Yale University School of Medicine, 333 Cedar Street, 1074 LMP, PO. Box 208030, New Haven, CT 06520-8030, USA
[b] Department of Dermatology and Skin Science, University of British Columbia, 835 West 10th Avenue, Vancouver, BC V5Z 4E8, Canada
[c] Department of Dermatology, Northwestern University Feinberg School of Medicine, 676 North Saint Clair Street, Suite 1600, Chicago, IL 60611, USA
* Corresponding author.
E-mail address: rkundu@nmff.org

Dermatol Clin 29 (2011) 111–123
doi:10.1016/j.det.2010.08.010

Table 1
Adverse effects of skin lightening compounds

Hydroquinone	Mercurials	Topical Corticosteroids
Allergic contact dermatitis	Allergic contact dermatitis	Allergic contact dermatitis
Hyperpigmentation	Hyperpigmentation	Skin atrophy/striae atrophica
Corneal melanosis/ degeneration	Anxiety/depression/psychosis	Acne vulgaris/perioral dermatitis
Exogenous ochronosis	Erythroderma	Cellulitis/dermatophytosis
Conjunctival pigmentation	Acute tubular necrosis	Cataracts/glaucoma
Trimethylaminuria	Membranous nephropathy	Hypertrichosis
Impaired wound healing	Peripheral neuropathy	Rosacea/telangiectasia
Nail discoloration	Positive antinuclear antibody test	Adrenal suppression/Cushing syndrome
Squamous cell carcinoma?	Tremor	Squamous cell carcinoma?

black-haired cats, which was reversible after hydroquinone discontinuation. Shortly after, in 1941, Martin and Ansbacher[6] showed that hydroquinone ingestion induced graying of hair in mice. In the 1950s, hydroquinone was used as a sunscreen in the Southern United States, and users reported skin lightening as a complication.[7] Since 1956, hydroquinone has been available in various OTC formulations for skin lightening purposes in the United States.[8] In 1961, Spencer[9] reported the first clinical trial evaluating hydroquinone as a skin lightener, and since then hydroquinone has remained the preferred treatment for various hyperpigmentation disorders, such as melasma, PIH, and lentigines.

Topical Corticosteroids

TCs are subdivided according to strength (class I–VII), with class I (ie, clobetasol) being the most potent and class VII (ie, hydrocortisone) the least potent.[10] The strength of TCs is determined by the vasoconstriction assay, in which potency is associated with the degree of blood vessel blanching in the upper dermis.[10,11] TCs have long been used for their skin lightening properties and are often the most commonly used skin lighteners in Africa.[12,13] TCs are believed to bleach the skin through inhibiting pro-opiomelanocortin (POMC), the precursor protein for α-melanocyte-stimulating hormone (α-MSH), which is produced in the intermediate lobe of the pituitary to stimulate epidermal melanin production.[14]

Mercurials

Mercury exists in three forms: organic, inorganic, and elemental.[14] Mercury-containing creams and ointments have been used for centuries to treat infections (ie, syphilis),[15] impetigo,[16] phthiriasis (lice),[17] and inflammatory skin diseases (ie, psoriasis),[18] but more recently they have been used as skin lighteners.[8,14] Mercurials exert their skin lightening actions through inhibition of sulfhydryl enzymes or mercaptans,[3] ultimately resulting in suppression of tyrosinase (the rate-limiting enzyme in the melanin pathway) and decreased melanogenesis.[14]

ADVERSE EFFECTS OF TOPICAL SKIN LIGHTENING COMPOUNDS
Hydroquinone

Although hydroquinone is one of the most effective and popular skin lightening compounds, it has been shown to cause multiple cutaneous and systemic side effects.[1] The most common acute complication of hydroquinone use is irritant contact dermatitis (up to 70% of patients) (**Fig. 1**), followed by PIH, hypopigmentation, and allergic contact dermatitis.[1,19,20] Chronic complications of hydroquinone exposure include nail discoloration[21–23] or "pseudo yellow-nail syndrome,"[14] conjunctival pigmentation,[24] corneal melanosis and degeneration,[24–26] peripheral neuropathy,[27] decreased skin elasticity,[14] impaired wound healing,[14,28] and wound dehiscence,[14,28] particularly after abdominal procedures such as caesarian section or hysterectomy. Another unique complication of chronic hydroquinone use is trimethylaminuria or "fish odor syndrome,"[28,29] characterized by a rotten fish body odor caused by excretion of trimethylamine in the saliva, sweat, urine, and vagina.[30] An association between hydroquinone and squamous cell carcinoma has also been suggested, although all reported cases had a history of prior or concomitant TC use.[31,32] Further studies are needed to

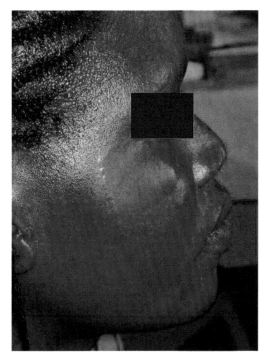

Fig. 1. A Senegalese woman with a peculiar reddish hue that some bleaching creams cause.

properly determine the risk of skin cancer in hydroquinone users.

The most severe and widely recognized complication of chronic hydroquinone use is exogenous ochronosis,[1,33] with at least 789 reported cases, 756 of which occurred in Africa.[34] Ochronosis can exist in both endogenous and exogenous form, the former associated with alkaptonuria, an autosomal recessive disorder (1:25,000) characterized by the absence of homogentisic acid oxidase (HGOA),[35] and the latter typically attributed to hydroquinone-containing compounds.[1,33] Exogenous ochronosis has also been associated with antimalarials,[36–38]; carbolic acid (phenol) leg ulcer compresses[39,40]; resorcinol[41]; mercury[42]; levodopa[43]; and picric acid.[42] In the inherited form, HGOA enzyme deficiency leads to homogentisic acid accumulation, which polymerizes to form ochre-colored pigments that deposit in the skin, cartilage, and tendons.[35,44] Alkaptonuria is classically characterized by the triad of painless cutaneous hyperpigmentation (ochronosis), arthritis, and homogentisic aciduria, in which urine turns black when left standing or on contact with air or an alkali.[35,44] Thickening of the cartilage of the pinnae, calcification of the aortic valve and prostate gland, and dark cerumen are also characteristic.[44] Although exogenous ochronosis is clinically and histologically similar to its endogenous form, it is not inherited and no systemic symptoms are observed.

The term *ochronosis* ("yellow disease" in Greek) was coined by Virchow[45] in 1866, when he described a patient whose cartilage appeared blue-black grossly, but was yellow-brown when viewed microscopically. In 1901, Pick[46] reported the first exogenous form of ochronosis in a patient with prolonged exposure to phenols. In 1975, Findlay and colleagues[33] described the first cases of hydroquinone-induced exogenous ochronosis in 35 South African Bantu women that used high-concentration (3.5%–7%) hydroquinone for several years. In 1979, Dogliotte and Liebowitz[47] classified exogenous ochronosis into three different stages: (1) erythema and mild pigmentation, (2) hyperpigmentation, black colloid milia, and scanty atrophy, and (3) papulonodules with or without surrounding inflammation. The first case in the United States of exogenous ochronosis caused by hydroquinone use was reported in 1983 by Cullison and colleagues,[48] which was followed with reports by Hoshaw and colleagues,[49] Connor and Braunstein,[50] and Lawrence and colleagues,[51] all in patients using low-concentration (≤3%) hydroquinone for a short duration (≤1 year). Although various theories exist regarding the pathogenesis of exogenous ochronosis, the most accepted is that of Penneys'[52] which attributes the condition to hydroquinone's inhibition of the enzyme HGOA, leading to the accumulation of homogentisic acid, which then polymerizes to form ochre pigments in the papillary dermis.

Exogenous ochronosis is characterized by gray-brown or blue-black macules coalescing into patches, which are occasionally accompanied by pinpoint, dark brown, caviar-like papules.[33,47,53] Exogenous ochronosis is typically symmetrically distributed in photoexposed areas, particularly over osseous surfaces in the infraorbital and zygomatic regions,[33] leading some to speculate that ultraviolet exposure might be a risk factor.[54] Histologically, exogenous ochronosis is characterized by normal epidermis, curved ochre-colored banana-shaped structures in the papillary dermis, dermal solar elastosis, and degeneration of collagen and elastic fibers.[1,33,48] Occasionally, sarcoid-like granulomas with multinucleated giant cells are seen surrounding the ochronotic particles.[38,48,49,55] On dermoscopy, blue-gray amorphous areas can be seen obliterating follicular openings.[53] The ochronotic pigment stains blue-black with methylene blue and black with Fontana stain; they do not stain with Prussian blue for iron.[50,56]

Several modalities have been experimentally used to treat exogenous ochronosis, but results have not been reassuring.[42] Some reports have noted improvement with carbon dioxide laser,[57] dermabrasion,[57,58] Q-switched ruby laser,[48] Q-switched alexandrite laser (755 nm),[59] tetracycline [60] and retinoic acid,[57,61] whereas cryotherapy and trichloroacetic acid have not shown efficacy.[57] Occasionally, hydroquinone discontinuation leads to reversal of the hyperpigmentation, but this can take up to several years.[33,48,49]

Topical Corticosteroids

Although TCs are frequently used as skin lightening agents,[12,13] they are associated with multiple dermatologic and systemic side effects.[8,14,28,62,63] Common cutaneous complications associated with TC application include acne vulgaris,[13,28,63] allergic contact dermatitis,[13,64,65] skin atrophy,[66—68] perioral dermatitis,[68] hypertrichosis,[28,63] rosacea,[14,28] striae atrophica,[13,28,63,67] and telangiectasias.[63,66] The skin on the neck seems particularly prone to atrophy, sometimes producing a rippled, "plucked chicken" appearance, otherwise known as pseudo-pseudoxanthoma elasticum.[14] Chronic periocular TC use can cause ophthalmologic complications, such as cataracts and glaucoma.[14] TC users are also particularly prone to developing infections such as cellulitis,[14] dermatophytosis,[13,28,63] erysipelas,[14,28] folliculitis,[14] and scabies.[13,28] Dermatophyte infections are especially common[14] and include tinea incognito,[14] widespread tinea corporis[14] and tinea faciei,[14] which can mimic roseacea[69] or lupus erythematosus.[70,71] Furthermore, chronic users are more likely to develop viral warts,[28] which tend to appear simultaneously on the neck and upper trunk, a finding that Olumide and colleagues[14] nicknamed the "pseudo Leser-Trélat sign."

TC use is also associated with various systemic complications such as hypothalamic-pituitary-adrenal (HPA) axis suppression, Cushing syndrome,[28,72,73] diabetes mellitus,[63] and hypertension.[74] The most worrisome of these complications is HPA dysfunction causing adrenal insufficiency,[10,72,75,76] which can be life-threatening. Adrenal suppression has long been regarded as a complication of high-dose TCs (ie, >50 g/wk of clobetasol propionate), but patients taking low doses (ie, 7.5 g/wk) have also experienced adrenal suppression.[77] In 2001, Perret and colleagues[78] assessed the functionality of the HPA axis among decade-long TC users in Sénégal and reported significantly lower plasma cortisol levels in response to cosyntropin stimulation compared with controls.

Another potential adverse effect from chronic daily use of a potent TC is "steroid addiction syndrome," which is characterized by intense burning and potentially permanent erythema due to withdrawal vasodilatation.[14] The irreversible form of pronounced erythema, often referred to as homme rouge, occurs more commonly in male users.[14]

Other less-common reactions reported with TC use include avascular necrosis of the femoral head[79] and squamous cell carcinoma.[31,32] Additionally, chronic use of TCs may mask other pathologic conditions, as was observed in a patient with leprosy.[80] The risk of these adverse reactions is potentiated when high-potency formulations are used on sites with fragile, thin skin (ie, face, armpit, groin) for prolonged periods or under occlusion, which promotes penetration.[10,14] Individuals particularly at risk for developing adrenal suppression include infants and patients with damaged skin barriers.[10]

Mercurials

Mercury-containing skin lightening agents or mercurials usually contain either mercury chloride or calomel and ammoniated mercury chloride, which are inorganic salts.[81] Mercury, as thimerosal, is also commonly used in the manufacturing of mascara and other cosmetics.[82] Acute or chronic exposure to topical mercury-containing compounds can cause dermatologic, renal, and neurologic toxicity.[16,81,82] Classically, mercury poisoning was associated with felt hat manufacturers, hence the name "mad hatters disease," or in patients treated for cutaneous disorders such as syphilis or impetigo. However, skin lightening products have also emerged as a major cause of mercury toxicity.[8,14,83,84]

Common cutaneous complications of mercury use include allergic contact dermatitis, flushing, erythroderma, purpura, gingivostomatitis, and nail discoloration.[16,82,85,86] Chronic use of mercurial skin lighteners can cause a paradoxic hyperpigmentation, which might be caused by dermal deposition of mercury-containing granules.[87] Mercury-induced neuropsychiatric toxicity includes metallic taste, tremor, peripheral neuropathy, erethism, memory loss, anxiety, depression, and psychosis.[16,84] Other complications include positive antinuclear antibody titers[88,89] and a suggested association with systemic lupus erythematosus (SLE),[90] as metallic mercury exposure has been shown to accelerate SLE development in lupus-prone mice.[91] Maternal use of mercury-containing soap during pregnancy has resulted in prenatal and postnatal intoxication, as mercury can cross the placenta.[16] In children, inorganic mercury exposure has also been associated with acrodynia.[16]

Nephrotoxicity is another potential complication related to mercury use.[83,88,92–96] In one report, 50% of young African women in Kenya who used mercury-containing skin lightening creams developed glomerular lesions.[92] The type of mercury-associated kidney injury depends on the form of mercury and the rate of administration.[83] Organic and metallic mercury are lipophilic and typically cause neurotoxicity, whereas inorganic mercury typically causes nephrotoxicity.[97] Still, any form of mercury can cause tubular or glomerular renal disease depending on the length of contact, with acute exposure usually causing tubular injury (acute tubular necrosis) and chronic exposure usually causing glomerular injury (membranous nephropathy, immune complex–mediated glomerulonephritis, minimal change disease).[83,88,92–96] Cole and colleagues[15] showed that the amount of mercury applied to the skin is proportional to the amount excreted by the kidneys. Still, mercury-induced membranous nephropathy typically resolves spontaneously after exposure cessation.[92]

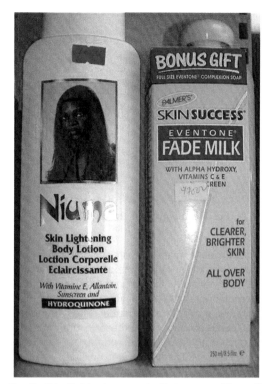

Fig. 2. Skin lightening agents that are readily available for sale in Ghana.

PSYCHOSOCIAL ASPECT

Although dermatologic disorders are not generally considered to be life-threatening, suicide has been reported in patients with "skin failure."[98–101] Psychodermatologic problems are more common in women, and facial symptomatology seems to be a particular risk factor for depression and suicidal ideations.[99] Disorders of pigmentation, such as melasma, vitiligo, PIH, lentigo, and idiopathic guttate hypomelanosis, are prevalent and have been shown to significantly impact health-related quality of life (HRQOL) in a deleterious manner.[102–104] A recent United States study showed that 80% of randomly selected patients at a private dermatology clinic had pigmentation disorders that significantly affected their quality of life.[104] Approximately 47.3% of patients felt self-conscious about their skin, 32.7% felt unattractive, and 23.6% felt their disorder affected their day-to-day activities, although few patients sought or received treatment for these conditions.[104] Treatment with skin lightening agents has been shown to improve these unfavorable psychosocial and HRQOL issues.[103]

The habitual use of skin lightening compounds has long been commonplace in Africa, particularly Ghana[31,105] (Fig. 2), Kenya,[92] Nigeria,[28,106]

Sénégal,[13] and Zimbabwe,[107] and in India,[108] but has recently become recognized in other parts of the world, including North America,[48,49] South America,[53] Central America,[109] Great Britain,[83] Europe,[110] Japan,[111] Southeast Asia[112] (Fig. 3), and the Middle East.[113,114] For more than 50 years, the mainstay of therapy for Black, White, Asian, Indian, and Hispanic individuals with hyperpigmentation disorders has been hydroquinone.[115] Although traditionally regarded as a female practice, men in Africa commonly use skin lighteners,[13] and recent articles suggest that they are becoming popular among men in India,[116] North America,[117] and Central America.[109]

Concerns regarding hydroquinone toxicity, particularly exogenous ochronosis and potential carcinogenicity, has led to rigid regulations in Africa, an OTC ban in Europe, abolishment in Japan, and a proposed OTC ban in the United States. Despite these concerns, human exposure to hydroquinone is common, because it is typically found in cosmetics,[118] cigarette smoke,[118] motor fuels and oils,[118] photograph developer,[118] and various foods, such as blueberries,[118] cranberries,[118] pears,[119] coffee,[119] tea,[119] and wheat products.[119] Still, no reports of malignancy associated with hydroquinone have been confirmed, and regulatory groups have determined that evidence

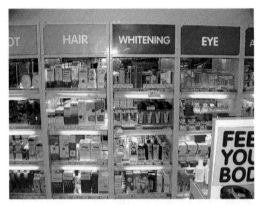

Fig. 3. Upscale pharmacy in Thailand.

is insufficient to classify hydroquinone as a carcinogen.[1] In fact, several large studies have shown that individuals with occupational exposure to hydroquinone have similar[120] or decreased[121,122] all-cause mortality and cancer rates compared with controls. Although excessive oral ingestion of photographic developer containing hydroquinone has been associated with suicide,[123] studies investigating intentional ingestion of hydroquinone in large quantities have reported no significant abnormalities.[25]

Africa

Use of skin lightening products is popular in Africa,[80] with an estimated prevalence of 25% to 96%.[12,67] In Sub-Saharan Africa, a desire to have lighter skin has been reported as a major motivating factor for using these products, as white skin is still associated with social privileges in certain communities.[28] Several prospective studies conducted in Dakar, Sénégal showed that skin lightening is most prevalent among dark-skinned, illiterate, working, married women between 30 to 44 years of age.[12] TCs and hydroquinone are the most frequently used lighteners, with joint hyperpigmentation, striae, and skin atrophy being the most commonly reported complications.[12,28]

In a dermatologic clinic in Lagos, Nigeria, 92% of women and 5% of men reported using skin lighteners, and most were not aware that skin pigment served a protective function.[28] A study conducted at a maternity clinic in Dakar, Sénégal by Mahe and colleagues[124] showed that 68.7% of pregnant women used skin lighteners, specifically hydroquinone and highly potent TCs, throughout their gestational period, some even reporting initiating or increasing use as a result of their pregnancy. Regarding pregnancy outcomes, no significant difference was noted between skin lighteners and controls, but users of highly potent TCs had lower plasma cortisol levels, smaller placentas, and a higher rate of low birthweight infants.[124] Application of these agents is of particular concern in Africa, where products are readily available without prescription and are used for prolonged periods. Percutaneous absorption is also enhanced in tropical climates because of the occlusive effect of heat and humidity.

Exogenous ochronosis from hydroquinone use is most commonly observed in Africans (>750 of the nearly 800 reported cases),[34] but has also been described in Americans,[48,49,51] Mexicans,[61] Brazilians,[53] Spaniards,[125] Asians,[112] and Arabs.[126] The high prevalence in Africa may be confounded by several factors, such as the widespread use of antimalarials in the area, which is also known to cause exogenous ochronosis; the lack of biopsies performed; and the reliance on clinical diagnosis.[8] Resorcinol is also often used simultaneously with hydroquinone to hasten lightening, and the synergistic effect of these agents may contribute to the increased incidence of exogenous ochronosis in Africa.[127] Furthermore, in South Africa, most OTC hydroquinone products are in the form of a penetrating enhancing vehicle (ie, hydroalcoholic lotion), which enhances cutaneous absorption.[128] After the study by Findlay and colleagues,[33] in 1980 the upper limit of hydroquinone in OTC skin lightening products in South Africa was reduced from 8% to 2%,[129] although no proper studies showed this concentration to be safe.[81]

India

Studies assessing the prevalence of skin lightening in India could not be found, although this practice accounts for approximately 61% (1000 crore rupees, $250 million) of the Indian dermatologic market.[108] The desire for lighter skin in India likely originated from the structure of Hinduism's social hierarchy, in which those belonging to higher castes typically had fairer complexions.[116] Furthermore, throughout its history, India has been invaded by lighter-skinned nations, such as Great Britain, and therefore fairness, strength, and supremacy have become interconnected.[116] Today, lighter skin is associated with superior status and beauty, as evidenced by newspaper matrimonial advertisements, in which fairness is considered a favorable factor for engagement.[108,116] Paradoxically, in a country fixated on attaining a fair complexion, depigmentation disorders, such as vitiligo, are socially stigmatized and hinder one's possibility for marriage.[108]

Although Indian women have used bleaching agents for decades, the skin lightening industry also has began targeting men recently.[116,130] Various television, newspaper, and Internet advertisements are attempting to convey the message that lighter skin makes men more attractive and successful. For example, to promote its male-directed line of skin lighteners, Vaseline recently released a Facebook skin-whitening application, "Vaseline Men: Be Prepared," inviting users to, "Transform your face on Facebook with Vaseline men," adding that their product "not only whitens your skin but is also designed to reduce five types of dark spots on your face."[130]

North America

No formal studies have assessed the prevalence of skin lightening in North America. According to the US Food and Drug Administration (FDA) Over-The-Counter Miscellaneous Panel, 2% hydroquinone has long been considered a safe concentration.[8] However, on August 29, 2006, the FDA proposed banning all OTC hydroquinone skin lightening agents that were not approved through the New Drug Application process.[8,34,115] This motion was stimulated by the increasing incidence of hydroquinone-induced exogenous ochronosis and other adverse drug reactions (most of which are reported in Africa), and several drug manufacturers' disregard of the FDA's request for hydroquinone safety studies.[8,34] The purpose of the proposal was to "establish that OTC skin bleaching drug products are not generally recognized as safe and effective (GRASE)," according to the Kefauver Harris Amendment, which was passed in 1962 to ensure that drugs demonstrated efficacy in addition to safety, a requirement included in the original Food, Drug and Cosmetics Act of 1938.[34,115] In March 2010, the FDA[131] announced that the National Toxicology Program would be conducting further studies on hydroquinone's potential for reproductive toxicity and dermal carcinogenicity in mice and rats.

Classically believed to only occur with use of high-concentration ($\geq3.5\%$) hydroquinone products used for prolonged periods (≥1 year),[53,132] exogenous ochronosis has also been reported with use of lower concentrations ($\leq3\%$)[48–51,53,61,125,133] and acute use (≤1 year).[48–51,61] Of the 22 cases of exogenous ochronosis reported in the United States, 21 were associated with low-concentration hydroquinone (1%–2%), generally used for prolonged periods (≥1 year).[34] Thus, the average number of exogenous ochronosis cases reported in the United States is approximately one per year, or 1 in 10

million tubes sold, leading some to disagree with the FDA, believing that hydroquinone's benefits outweigh its risks.[34]

In 1973, mercury-containing cosmetics were banned in the United States because of safety concerns but, despite this apparent prohibition, unregulated mercurials are still readily attainable without a prescription. In 1996, mercury poisoning associated with a skin lightening product, Creme de Belleza—Manning, which was produced in Mexico and illegally imported into the United States, was reported in more than 400 Mexican-American women in Arizona, California, New Mexico, and Texas.[134,135] Recently, toxicity associated with mercury-containing soap has been reported,[136] and an investigation of 50 skin lightening creams, most purchased OTC in Chicago stores and some online, detected unlawful amounts of mercury in 6 products.[137]

ALTERNATIVES TO TRADITIONAL SKIN LIGHTENING COMPOUNDS

The gold standard dermatologic agent for skin lightening has classically been hydroquinone, until regulatory agencies in Africa, Asia, Europe, and the United States questioned its safety profile. This scrutiny encouraged research into alternative agents to reduce skin pigmentation, such as aleosin, arbutin, azelaic acid, ascorbic acid, kojic acid, licorice extract, mequinol, N-acetyl glucosamine, soy proteins, and retinoids[138] (Table 2). The three primary prescription alternatives to hydroquinone are mequinol (4-hydroxyanisole), often in combination with 0.01% tretinoin and vitamin C (ascorbic acid)[138]; azelaic acid,[138,139] which is derived from Pityrosporum ovale cultures; and retinoids, in the form of adapalene, tazarotene, and

Table 2	
Alternative skin lightening agents	
Skin Lighteners	**Mechanism of Action**
Aleosin	Tyrosinase inhibition
Arbutin	Tyrosinase inhibition
Azelaic acid	Tyrosinase inhibition
Ascorbic acid	Melanogenesis inhibition
Kojic acid	Tyrosinase inhibition
Licorice extract	Melanogenesis inhibition
Mequinol	Tyrosinase inhibition
N-acetyl glucosamine	Tyrosinase glycosylation inhibition
Retinoids	Melanogenesis inhibition
Soy extract	Melanosome transfer inhibition

tretinoin.[138,140] The most effective OTC alternatives to hydroquinone are arbutin,[141] extracted from the leaves of the bear-berry plant; its synthetic and more efficacious form, deoxyarbutin[142]; and kojic acid,[143] which is obtained from Aspergillus and Penicillium cultures. Other less-effective, but safer OTC alternative agents include licorice extract (liquiritin)[144]; soybean extract (soybean trypsin inhibitor [STI])[145]; N-acetyl glucosamine[146]; aleosin,[147] derived from the aloe vera plant and often combined with arbutin or deoxyarbutin to enhance effectiveness[138]; and ascorbic acid,[148] which is typically ineffective unless used in combination with licorice extract, retinoids, or STI.[138] Given the questionable toxicity of currently popular skin lighteners on the market, further investigations into effective alternative agents with enhanced safety profiles are necessary.

Due to potential for various cutaneous and systemic complications associated with mono-therapeutic skin lightening agents, combination compounds have been manufactured to reduce toxicity and improve effectiveness. In 2002, a triple-combination cream composed of 4% hydroquinone, 0.01% fluocinolone acetonide (class VI low-potency TC), and 0.05% tretinoin or retinoic acid (Tri-Luma) was FDA-approved for the treatment of melasma. Once-daily application of this triple-combination therapy (TCT) was shown to be more effective for treating melasma than monotherapies (4% hydroquinone applied twice daily)[149,150] and dual therapies (hydroquinone + retinoic acid; hydroquinone + fluocinolone acetonide; or fluocinolone acetonide + retinoic acid).[104] Compared with hydroquinone alone, TCT was associated with superior patient satisfaction,[149] enhanced self-perception,[151] overall quality of life improvement,[152] and improved cost-effectiveness,[126,150] as well as a comparable safety profile.[104,149,150,152]

Furthermore, TC-induced skin atrophy has been minimal in patients using combination creams, possibly because of tretinoin, which seems to act as a protective factor by promoting dermal collagen synthesis and epidermal growth without lessening the anti-inflammatory effect.[153] Incidence of adverse events have varied among studies, with similar[104,150] and worse[149] safety profiles reported with TCT, although all complications have been mild, with no reports of severe side effects. The most commonly reported adverse effects associated with TCT are erythema, burning, and desquamation, with few reports of minor atrophy and no reports of exogenous ochronosis.[104,149,150,154] Two cases of skin atrophy related to TCT use have been reported, although

reactions were mild and did not lead to treatment discontinuation.[154] Therefore, TCT seems to be effective and exhibits a safe profile with low potential for adverse events.

SUMMARY

Given the widespread use of topical skin lightening compounds, practicing dermatologists must be aware of their current clinical indications and potential adverse effects. Dermatologists should also be able to differentiate melasma from hydroquinone-induced exogenous ochronosis, because these conditions are often confused. Prescriptions for skin lightening products should be precise in terms of concentration, amount to apply, and duration of treatment. Furthermore, patients should be provided with information regarding potential adverse effects, such as exogenous ochronosis or skin atrophy, and potentiation of these toxicities if multiple lightening agents are used simultaneously. If any of the aforementioned severe effects occur, the offending agent should be discontinued and, if treatment is still necessary, an alternative prescribed, such as mequinol or azelaic acid. Further studies investigating the prevalence of skin lightener use, motivating factors, and complications are warranted in the United States, India, and other countries where skin bleaching is practiced.

ACKNOWLEDGMENTS

The authors kindly acknowledge Dr Scott Norton for the generous contribution of his photographs.

REFERENCES

1. Nordlund JJ, Grimes PE, Ortonne JP. The safety of hydroquinone. J Eur Acad Dermatol Venereol 2006; 20(7):781–7.
2. Jimbow K, Obata H, Pathak MA, et al. Mechanism of depigmentation by hydroquinone. J Invest Dermatol 1974;62(4):436–49.
3. Denton CR, Lerner AB, Fitzpatrick TB. Inhibition of melanin formation by chemical agents. J Invest Dermatol 1952;18(2):119–35.
4. Barber ED, Hill T, Schum DB. The percutaneous absorption of hydroquinone (HQ) through rat and human skin in vitro. Toxicol Lett 1995;80(1–3): 167–72.
5. Oettel H. Hydroquinone poisoning. Arch Exp Pathol Pharmacol 1956;183:319–62.
6. Martin GJ, Ansbacher S. Confirmatory evidence of the chromotrichal activity of p-aminobenzoic acid. J Biol Chem 1941;13:441.

7. Denton CR. Skin protective agents. Med Bull (Ann Arbor) 1952;18(5):143–52.

8. Dadzie OE, Petit A. Skin bleaching: highlighting the misuse of cutaneous depigmenting agents. J Eur Acad Dermatol Venereol 2009;23(7): 741–50.

9. Spencer MC. Hydroquinone bleaching. Arch Dermatol 1961;84:181–2.

10. Levin C, Maibach HI. Topical corticosteroid-induced adrenocortical insufficiency: clinical implications. Am J Clin Dermatol 2002;3(3):141–7.

11. McKenzie AW, Stoughton RB. Method for comparing percutaneous absorption of steroids. Arch Dermatol 1962;86:608–10.

12. Wone I, Tal-Dia A, Diallo OF, et al. Prevalence of the use of skin bleaching cosmetics in two areas in Dakar (Senegal). Dakar Med 2000;45(2):154–7 [in French].

13. Mahe A, Ly F, Aymard G, et al. Skin diseases associated with the cosmetic use of bleaching products in women from Dakar, Senegal. Br J Dermatol 2003;148(3):493–500.

14. Olumide YM, Akinkugbe AO, Altraide D, et al. Complications of chronic use of skin lightening cosmetics. Int J Dermatol 2008;47(4):344–53.

15. Cole HN, Shreiber MA, Sollman T. Mercurial ointments in the treatment of syphilis. Arch Derm Syphilol 1930;21(3):372–93.

16. Engler DE. Mercury "bleaching" creams. J Am Acad Dermatol 2005;52(6):1113–4.

17. Vena GA, Foti C, Grandolfo M, et al. Mercury exanthem. Contact Dermatitis 1994;31(4):214–6.

18. Gordon B, Inman PM, Trinder P. Mercury absorption and psoriasis. Br Med J 1956;2(5003): 1202–6.

19. Balina LM, Graupe K. The treatment of melasma. 20% azelaic acid versus 4% hydroquinone cream. Int J Dermatol 1991;30(12):893–5.

20. Grimes PE. A microsponge formulation of hydroquinone 4% and retinol 0.15% in the treatment of melasma and postinflammatory hyperpigmentation. Cutis 2004;74(6):362–8.

21. Garcia RL, White JW Jr, Willis WF. Hydroquinone nail pigmentation. Arch Dermatol 1978;114(9): 1402–3.

22. Arndt KA, Fitzpatrick TB. Topical use of hydroquinone as a depigmenting agent. JAMA 1965; 194(9):965–7.

23. Mann RJ, Harman RR. Nail staining due to hydroquinone skin-lightening creams. Br J Dermatol 1983;108(3):363–5.

24. Anderson B. Corneal and conjunctival pigmentation among workers engaged in manufacture of hydroquinone. Arch Ophthal 1947;38(6):812–26.

25. DeCaprio AP. The toxicology of hydroquinone—relevance to occupational and environmental exposure. Crit Rev Toxicol 1999;29(3):283–330.

26. Naumann G. Corneal damage in hydroquinone workers. A clinicopathologic study. Arch Ophthalmol 1966;76(2):189–94.

27. Karamagi C, Owino E, Katabira ET. Hydroquinone neuropathy following use of skin bleaching creams: case report. East Afr Med J 2001;78(4):223–4.

28. Ajose FO. Consequences of skin bleaching in Nigerian men and women. Int J Dermatol 2005; 44(Suppl 1):41–3.

29. Jordaan HF, Van Niekerk DJ. Transepidermal elimination in exogenous ochronosis. A report of two cases. Am J Dermatopathol 1991;13(4):418–24.

30. Ruocco V, Florio M. Fish-odor syndrome: an olfactory diagnosis. Int J Dermatol 1995;34(2):92–3.

31. Addo H. Squamous cell carcinoma associated with prolonged bleaching. Ghana Med J 2000;34:3.

32. Ly F, Kane A, Deme A, et al. First cases of squamous cell carcinoma associated with cosmetic use of bleaching compounds. Ann Dermatol Venereol 2010;137(2):128–31 [in French].

33. Findlay GH, Morrison JG, Simson IW. Exogenous ochronosis and pigmented colloid milium from hydroquinone bleaching creams. Br J Dermatol 1975;93(6):613–22.

34. Levitt J. The safety of hydroquinone: a dermatologist's response to the 2006 Federal Register. J Am Acad Dermatol 2007;57(5):854–72.

35. Phornphutkul C, Introne WJ, Perry MB, et al. Natural history of alkaptonuria. N Engl J Med 2002;347(26):2111–21.

36. Ludwig GD, Toole JF, Wood JC. Ochronosis from Quinacrine (Atabrine). Ann Intern Med 1963;59: 378–84.

37. Adler I, Klocker H, Oettel HJ, et al. [Problem of the liver function tests in the acute and chronic liver diseases]. Arztl Wochensch 1953;8(16):393–6 [in German].

38. Bruce S, Tschen JA, Chow D. Exogenous ochronosis resulting from quinine injections. J Am Acad Dermatol 1986;15(2 Pt 2):357–61 [in German].

39. Berry JL, PeatOchronosis S. Report of a case with carboluria. Lancet 1931;2:124–6.

40. Brogren N. Case of exogenetic ochronosis from carbolic acid compresses. Acta Derm Venereol 1952;32(3):258–60.

41. Thomas AE, Gisburn MA. Exogenous ochronosis and myxoedema from resorcinol. Br J Dermatol 1961;73:378–81.

42. Levin CY, Maibach H. Exogenous ochronosis. An update on clinical features, causative agents and treatment options. Am J Clin Dermatol 2001;2(4):213–7.

43. Kaufmann B, Wegmann W. Exogenous ochronosis after L-dopa treatment. Pathologe 1992;13(3): 164–6 [in German].

44. Van Offel JF, De Clerck LS, Francx LM, et al. The clinical manifestations of ochronosis: a review. Acta Clin Belg 1995;50(6):358–62.

45. Virchow R. Ein Fall von allgemeiner Ochronose der Knorpel und knorpelahnlichen Theile. Arch Pathol Anat Physiol 1866;37:212–9 [in German].

46. Pick L. Uber die ochronosis klin. Wochenschr 1906;43:478–80 [in German].

47. Dogliotte M, Leibowitz M. Granulomatous ochronosis—a cosmetic-induced skin disorder in blacks. S Afr Med J 1979;56:757–60.

48. Cullison D, Abele DC, O'Quinn JL. Localized exogenous ochronosis. J Am Acad Dermatol 1983;8(6): 882–9.

49. Hoshaw RA, Zimmerman KG, Menter A. Ochronosislike pigmentation from hydroquinone bleaching creams in American blacks. Arch Dermatol 1985; 121(1):105–8.

50. Connor T, Braunstein B. Hyperpigmentation following the use of bleaching creams. Localized exogenous ochronosis. Arch Dermatol 1987; 123(1):105–6, 108.

51. Lawrence N, Bligard CA, Reed R, et al. Exogenous ochronosis in the United States. J Am Acad Dermatol 1988;18(5 Pt 2):1207–11.

52. Penneys NS. Ochronosislike pigmentation from hydroquinone bleaching creams. Arch Dermatol 1985;121(10):1239–40.

53. Charlin R, Barcaui CB, Kac BK, et al. Hydroquinone-induced exogenous ochronosis: a report of four cases and usefulness of dermoscopy. Int J Dermatol 2008;47(1):19–23.

54. O'Donoghue MN, Lynfield YL, Derbes V. Ochronosis due to hydroquinone. J Am Acad Dermatol 1983;8(1):123.

55. Jacyk WK. Annular granulomatous lesions in exogenous ochronosis are manifestation of sarcoidosis. Am J Dermatopathol 1995;17(1):18–22.

56. Tidman MJ, Horton JJ, MacDonald DM. Hydroquinone-induced ochronosis—light and electronmicroscopic features. Clin Exp Dermatol 1986;11(3): 224–8.

57. Diven DG, Smith EB, Pupo RA, et al. Hydroquinone-induced localized exogenous ochronosis treated with dermabrasion and CO2 laser. J Dermatol Surg Oncol 1990;16(11):1018–22.

58. Lang PG Jr. Probable coexisting exogenous ochronosis and mercurial pigmentation managed by dermabrasion. J Am Acad Dermatol 1988; 19(5 Pt 2):942–6.

59. Bellew SG, Alster TS. Treatment of exogenous ochronosis with a Q-switched alexandrite (755 nm) laser. Dermatol Surg 2004;30(4 Pt 1): 555–8.

60. Fisher AA. Tetracycline treatment for sarcoid-like ochronosis due to hydroquinone. Cutis 1988; 42(1):19–20.

61. Howard KL, Furner BB. Exogenous ochronosis in a Mexican-American woman. Cutis 1990;45(3): 180–2.

62. Ly F. Skin diseases associated with the use of skin-bleaching products in Africa. Ann Dermatol Venereol 2006;133(11):899–906 [in French].

63. Nnoruka E, Okoye O. Topical steroid abuse: its use as a depigmenting agent. J Natl Med Assoc 2006; 98(6):934–9.

64. Boyle J, Peachey RD. Allergic contact dermatitis to Dermovate and Eumovate. Contact Dermatitis 1984;11(1):50–1.

65. Lutz ME, el-Azhary RA. Allergic contact dermatitis due to topical application of corticosteroids: review and clinical implications. Mayo Clin Proc 1997; 72(12):1141–4.

66. Keane FM, Munn SE, Taylor NF, et al. Unregulated use of clobetasol propionate. Br J Dermatol 2001; 144(5):1095–6.

67. Ly F, Soko AS, Dione DA, et al. Aesthetic problems associated with the cosmetic use of bleaching products. Int J Dermatol 2007;46(Suppl 1):15–7.

68. Otley CC, Sober A. Over-the-counter clobetasol propionate. Arch Dermatol 1994;130(1):121.

69. Lee SJ, Choi HJ, Hann SK. Rosacea-like tinea faciei. Int J Dermatol 1999;38(6):479–80.

70. Meymandi S, Wiseman MC, Crawford RI. Tinea faciei mimicking cutaneous lupus erythematosus: a histopathologic case report. J Am Acad Dermatol 2003;48(Suppl 2):S7–8.

71. Singh R, Bharu K, Ghazali W, et al. Tinea faciei mimicking lupus erythematosus. Cutis 1994;53(6): 297–8.

72. Staughton RC, August PJ. Cushing's syndrome and pituitary-adrenal suppression due to clobetasol propionate. Br Med J 1975;2(5968):419–21.

73. May P, Stein EJ, Ryter RJ, et al. Cushing syndrome from percutaneous absorption of triamcinolone cream. Arch Intern Med 1976;136(5):612–3.

74. Bwomda P, Sermijn E, Lacor P, et al. Glucocorticoid hypertension due to the use of bleaching skin cream, a case report. Acta Clin Belg 2005;60(3): 146–9.

75. Tobin AM, Barragry J, Kirby B, et al. Adrenal suppression following topical use of clobetasol propionate illegally supplied as a bleaching agent. Ir Med J 2005;98(4):118.

76. Gilbertson EO, Spellman MC, Piacquadio DJ, et al. Super potent topical corticosteroid use associated with adrenal suppression: clinical considerations. J Am Acad Dermatol 1998;38(2 Pt 2):318–21.

77. Ohman EM, Rogers S, Meenan FO, et al. Adrenal suppression following low-dose topical clobetasol propionate. J R Soc Med 1987;80(7):422–4.

78. Perret JL, Sane M, Gning S, et al. Hypothalamo-hypophyseal-adrenal hypofunction caused by the use of bleaching cosmetics in Senegal. Bull Soc Pathol Exot 2001;94(3):249–52 [in French].

79. Hogan DJ, Sibley JT, Lane PR. Avascular necrosis of the hips following longterm use of clobetasol

propionate. J Am Acad Dermatol 1986;14(3): 515–7.

80. Mahe A, Ly F, Badiane C, et al. Irrational use of skin-bleaching products can delay the diagnosis of leprosy. Int J Lepr Other Mycobact Dis 2002; 70(2):119–21.

81. Mire A. Skin-bleaching: poison, beauty, power, and the politics of the colour line. Resour Fem Res 2001;28(3–4):13–38.

82. de la Cuadra J. Cutaneous sensitivity to mercury and its compounds. Ann Dermatol Venereol 1993; 120(1):37–42 [in French].

83. Oliveira DB, Foster G, Savill J, et al. Membranous nephropathy caused by mercury-containing skin lightening cream. Postgrad Med J 1987;63(738): 303–4.

84. Saffer D, Tayob H, Bill PL, et al. Continued marketing of skin-lightening preparations containing mercury. S Afr Med J 1976;50(39):1499.

85. Alexander AMK. Chronishe Quecksilbervertifang durch langdauernden Gebrauch einer Sommersprossensalbe. Dtsch Med Wochenschr 1923;49: 1021 [in German].

86. Bockers M, Wagner R, Oster O. Nail dyschromia as the leading symptom in chronic mercury poisoning caused by a cosmetic bleaching preparation [in German]. Z Hautkr 1985;60(10):821–9.

87. Goeckermann W. A peculiar discolouration of the skin. JAMA 1975;84:506–7.

88. Tang HL, Chu KH, Mak YF, et al. Minimal change disease following exposure to mercury-containing skin lightening cream. Hong Kong Med J 2006; 12(4):316–8.

89. Silva IA, Nyland JF, Gorman A, et al. Mercury exposure, malaria, and serum antinuclear/antinucleolar antibodies in Amazon populations in Brazil: a cross-sectional study. Environ Health 2004;3(1):11.

90. Cooper GS, Parks CG, Treadwell EL, et al. Occupational risk factors for the development of systemic lupus erythematosus. J Rheumatol 2004; 31(10):1928–33.

91. Pollard KM, Pearson DL, Hultman P, et al. Xenobiotic acceleration of idiopathic systemic autoimmunity in lupus-prone bxsb mice. Environ Health Perspect 2001;109(1):27–33.

92. Barr RD, Rees PH, Cordy PE, et al. Nephrotic syndrome in adult Africans in Nairobi. Br Med J 1972;2(5806):131–4.

93. Barr RD. The mercurial nephrotic syndrome. East Afr Med J 1990;67(6):381–6.

94. Soo YO, Chow KM, Lam CW, et al. A whitened face woman with nephrotic syndrome. Am J Kidney Dis 2003;41(1):250–3.

95. Tubbs RR, Gephardt GN, McMahon JT, et al. Membranous glomerulonephritis associated with industrial mercury exposure. Study of pathogenetic mechanisms. Am J Clin Pathol 1982;77(4):409–13.

96. Kibukamusoke JW, Davies DR, Hutt MS. Membranous nephropathy due to skin-lightening cream. Br Med J 1974;2(5920):646–7.

97. Magos L. Mercury and mercurials. Br Med Bull 1975;31(3):241–5.

98. Monk BE, Rao YJ. Delusions of parasitosis with fatal outcome. Clin Exp Dermatol 1994;19(4): 341–2.

99. Cotterill JA. Dermatological non-disease: a common and potentially fatal disturbance of cutaneous body image. Br J Dermatol 1981; 104(6):611–9.

100. Cotterill J. Skin and the psyche. Proc R Coll Physicians Edinb 1995;25:29–33.

101. Cotterill JA, Cunliffe WJ. Suicide in dermatological patients. Br J Dermatol 1997;137(2):246–50.

102. Pawaskar MD, Parikh P, Markowski T, et al. Melasma and its impact on health-related quality of life in Hispanic women. J Dermatolog Treat 2007;18(1): 5–9.

103. Balkrishnan R, Kelly AP, McMichael A, et al. Improved quality of life with effective treatment of facial melasma: the pigment trial. J Drugs Dermatol 2004;3(4):377–81.

104. Taylor A, Pawaskar M, Taylor SL, et al. Prevalence of pigmentary disorders and their impact on quality of life: a prospective cohort study. J Cosmet Dermatol 2008;7(3):164–8.

105. Addo H. A clinical study of hydroquinone reaction in skin bleaching in Ghana. Ghana Med J 1992; 26:448–53.

106. Adebajo SB. An epidemiological survey of the use of cosmetic skin lightening cosmetics among traders in Lagos, Nigeria. West Afr J Med 2002; 21(1):51–5.

107. Muchadeyi E, Thompson S, Baker N. A survey of the constituents, availability and use of skin lightening creams in Zimbabwe. Cent Afr J Med 1983; 29(11):225–7.

108. Verma SB. Obsession with light skin-shedding some light on use of skin lightening products in India. Int J Dermatol 2010;49(4):464–5.

109. Pichardo R, Vallejos Q, Feldman SR, et al. The prevalence of melasma and its association with quality of life in adult male Latino migrant workers. Int J Dermatol 2009;48(1):22–6.

110. Petit A, Cohen-Ludmann C, Clevenbergh P, et al. Skin lightening and its complications among African people living in Paris. J Am Acad Dermatol 2006;55(5):873–8.

111. Ashikari M. Cultivating Japanese whiteness: the 'whitening' cosmetics boom and the Japanese identity. J Mater Cult 2005;10:73–91.

112. Tan SK, Sim CS, Goh CL. Hydroquinone-induced exogenous ochronosis in Chinese—two case reports and a review. Int J Dermatol 2008;47(6): 639–40.

113. al-Saleh I, al-Doush I. Mercury content in skin-lightening creams and potential hazards to the health of Saudi women. J Toxicol Environ Health 1997;51(2):123–30.

114. Hamed SH, Tayyem R, Nimer N, et al. Skin-lightening practice among women living in Jordan: prevalence, determinants, and user's awareness. Int J Dermatol 2010;49(4):414–20.

115. Toombs EL. Hydroquinone—what is its future? Dermatol Ther 2007;20(3):149–56.

116. Radio NPR. In India, Skin-whitening creams reflect old biases. 2009. Available at: http://www.npr.org/templates/story/story.php?storyId=120340646. Accessed August 20, 2010.

117. Saint Louis C. Creams offering lighter skin may bring risks. 2000. Available at: http://www.nytimes.com/2010/01/16/health/16skin.html. Accessed June 1, 2010.

118. Hydroquinone IARC. Monogr Eval Carcinog Risks Hum 1999;71:691–719.

119. Deisinger PJ, Hill TS, English JC. Human exposure to naturally occurring hydroquinone. J Toxicol Environ Health 1996;47(1):31–46.

120. Friedlander BR, Hearne FT, Newman BJ. Mortality, cancer incidence, and sickness—absence in photographic processors: an epidemiologic study. J Occup Med 1982;24(8):605–13.

121. Pifer JW, Hearne FT, Friedlander BR, et al. Mortality study of men employed at a large chemical plant, 1972 through 1982. J Occup Med 1986;28(6):438–44.

122. Pifer JW, Hearne FT, Swanson FA, et al. Mortality study of employees engaged in the manufacture and use of hydroquinone. Int Arch Occup Environ Health 1995;67(4):267–80.

123. Saito T, Takeichi S. Experimental studies on the toxicity of lithographic developer solution. J Toxicol Clin Toxicol 1995;33(4):343–8.

124. Mahe A, Perret JL, Ly F, et al. The cosmetic use of skin-lightening products during pregnancy in Dakar, Senegal: a common and potentially hazardous practice. Trans R Soc Trop Med Hyg 2007;101(2):183–7.

125. Huerta BM, Sanchez VM. Exogenous ochronosis. J Drugs Dermatol 2006;5(1):80–1.

126. Alikhan A, Daly M, Wu J, et al. Cost-effectiveness of a hydroquinone/tretinoin/fluocinolone acetonide cream combination in treating melasma in the United States. J Dermatolog Treat 2010;21(5):276–81.

127. Burke P, Maibach H. Exogenous ochronosis: an overview. J Dermatolog Treat 1997;8:21–6.

128. Bucks DA, McMaster JR, Guy RH, et al. Percutaneous absorption of hydroquinone in humans: effect of 1-dodecylazacycloheptan-2-one (azone) and the 2-ethylhexyl ester of 4-(dimethylamino) benzoic acid (Escalol 507). J Toxicol Environ Health 1988;24(3):279–89.

129. Hardwick N, Van Gelder LW, Van der Merwe CA, et al. Exogenous ochronosis: an epidemiological study. Br J Dermatol 1989;120(2):229–38.

130. Whiteman H. Vaseline skin-lightening app stirs debate. 2010. Available at: http://edition.cnn.com/2010/WORLD/asiapcf/07/16/facebook.skin.lightening.app/#fbid=mmipxRqFmFQ. Accessed July 20, 2010.

131. FDA. Hydroquinone studies under the national toxicology program (NTP). 2010. Available at: http://www.fda.gov/AboutFDA/CentersOffices/CDER/ucm203112.htm. Accessed July 15, 2010.

132. Findlay GH. Ochronosis following skin bleaching with hydroquinone. J Am Acad Dermatol 1982;6(6):1092–3.

133. Bongiorno MR, Arico M. Exogenous ochronosis and striae atrophicae following the use of bleaching creams. Int J Dermatol 2005;44(2):112–5.

134. Centers for Disease Control and Prevention (CDC). Update: mercury poisoning associated with beauty cream—Arizona, California, New Mexico, and Texas, 1996. MMWR Morb Mortal Wkly Rep 1996;45(29):633–5.

135. Centers for Disease Control and Prevention (CDC). Mercury poisoning associated with beauty cream—Texas, New Mexico, and California, 1995–1996. MMWR Morb Mortal Wkly Rep 1996;45(19):400–3.

136. Harada M, Nakachi S, Tasaka K, et al. Wide use of skin-lightening soap may cause mercury poisoning in Kenya. Sci Total Environ 2001;269(1–3):183–7.

137. Gabler E, Roe S. Some skin whitening creams contain toxic mercury, testing finds. 2010. Available at: http://www.chicagotribune.com/health/ct–met–mercury–skin–creams–20100518,0,4522094.story. Accessed July 20, 2010.

138. Draelos ZD. Skin lightening preparations and the hydroquinone controversy. Dermatol Ther 2007;20(5):308–13.

139. Fitton A, Goa KL. Azelaic acid. A review of its pharmacological properties and therapeutic efficacy in acne and hyperpigmentary skin disorders. Drugs 1991;41(5):780–98.

140. Kimbrough-Green CK, Griffiths CE, Finkel LJ, et al. Topical retinoic acid (tretinoin) for melasma in black patients. A vehicle-controlled clinical trial. Arch Dermatol 1994;130(6):727–33.

141. Hori I, Nihei K, Kubo I. Structural criteria for depigmenting mechanism of arbutin. Phytother Res 2004;18(6):475–9.

142. Boissy RE, Visscher M, DeLong MA. DeoxyArbutin: a novel reversible tyrosinase inhibitor with effective in vivo skin lightening potency. Exp Dermatol 2005;14(8):601–8.

143. Lim JT. Treatment of melasma using kojic acid in a gel containing hydroquinone and glycolic acid. Dermatol Surg 1999;25(4):282–4.

144. Amer M, Metwalli M. Topical liquiritin improves melasma. Int J Dermatol 2000;39(4):299–301.

145. Paine C, Sharlow E, Liebel F, et al. An alternative approach to depigmentation by soybean extracts via inhibition of the PAR-2 pathway. J Invest Dermatol 2001;116(4):587–95.

146. Bissett DL, Miyamoto K, Sun P, et al. Topical niacinamide reduces yellowing, wrinkling, red blotchiness, and hyperpigmented spots in aging facial skin. Int J Cosmet Sci 2004;26(5):231–8.

147. Choi S, Lee SK, Kim JE, et al. Aloesin inhibits hyperpigmentation induced by UV radiation. Clin Exp Dermatol 2002;27(6):513–5.

148. Espinal-Perez LE, Moncada B, Castanedo-Cazares JP. A double-blind randomized trial of 5% ascorbic acid vs. 4% hydroquinone in melasma. Int J Dermatol 2004;43(8):604–7.

149. Chan R, Park KC, Lee MH, et al. A randomized controlled trial of the efficacy and safety of a fixed triple combination (fluocinolone acetonide 0.01%, hydroquinone 4%, tretinoin 0.05%) compared with hydroquinone 4% cream in Asian patients with moderate to severe melasma. Br J Dermatol 2008;159(3):697–703.

150. Cestari T, Adjadj L, Hux M, et al. Cost-effectiveness of a fixed combination of hydroquinone/tretinoin/fluocinolone cream compared with hydroquinone alone in the treatment of melasma. J Drugs Dermatol 2007;6(2):153–60.

151. Rendon MI. Utilizing combination therapy to optimize melasma outcomes. J Drugs Dermatol 2004;3(Suppl 5):S27–34.

152. Cestari TF, Hexsel D, Viegas ML, et al. Validation of a melasma quality of life questionnaire for Brazilian Portuguese language: the MelasQoL-BP study and improvement of QoL of melasma patients after triple combination therapy. Br J Dermatol 2006;156(Suppl 1):13–20.

153. Kligman LH, Schwartz E, Lesnik RH, et al. Topical tretinoin prevents corticosteroid-induced atrophy without lessening the anti-inflammatory effect. Curr Probl Dermatol 1993;21:79–88.

154. Torok H, Taylor S, Baumann L, et al. A large 12-month extension study of an 8-week trial to evaluate the safety and efficacy of triple combination (TC) cream in melasma patients previously treated with TC cream or one of its dyads. J Drugs Dermatol 2005;4(5):592–7.

Human Immunodeficiency Virus and Leprosy: An Update

Diana N.J. Lockwood, MD, FRCP*, Saba M. Lambert, MBBS

KEYWORDS

- Human immunodeficiency virus • Leprosy • Coinfection
- Antiretroviral treatment

Co-infection with HIV has a major effect on the natural history of many diseases, particularly mycobacterial diseases. Early in the HIV epidemic it was predicted that HIV infections would worsen outcomes in leprosy patients with more patients developing lepromatous disease and patients having fewer immune reactions. Now that many patients receive HAART tuberculoid leprosy types predominate and reactions are an important clinical feature in co-infected patients.[1–4]

Leprosy is a chronic infectious disease affecting nerves and skin. It has a long incubation period of 2 to 10 years, and presents with a clinical spectrum depending on the relationship between the host immune system and the bacteria. At one end of the spectrum is tuberculoid leprosy, characterized by strong cell-mediated immunity (CMI) toward M leprae. These patients have few hypopigmented, anesthetic lesions. At the other pole is lepromatous leprosy (LL), which is characterized by the absence of a CMI response. These patients have numerous lesions and high bacillary loads. Most patients have features between these two extreme groups and fall in the categories of borderline tuberculous (BT), borderline borderline (BB) or borderline lepromatous (BL). The borderline cases are immunologically unstable and at greater risk of type 1 reaction, which affects mainly the nerves and skin. The lepromatous types of BL and LL are at higher risk of erythema nodosum leprosum (ENL), a more systemic and severe immunologic complication.

In 2008, 121 countries reported a total of 249,007 new leprosy cases to the World Health Organization (WHO). Most endemic countries for leprosy also have a high HIV prevalence, increasing the possibility of HIV–leprosy coinfection.

The few published small studies provide limited data on the course of leprosy in coinfected patients. HIV incidence was not found to be increased among leprosy patients compared with nonleprosy groups.[5,6] All types of leprosy can occur in coinfected patients. Two East African studies reporting an increase multibacillary (MB) cases.[7,8] However since the introduction of HAART borderline tuberculoid leprosy is the predominant form, as reported in Brazilian studies.[9,10] Coinfected patients treated with standard length WHO-multi-drug therapy (MDT), have responded adequately, although there might be a possibility of an increased relapse rate.[11] A Ugandan study demonstrated an increased risk of developing type 1 reactions in an MB leprosy patient with HIV,[12] and increased recurrence rates of type 1 reactions were seen in an Ethiopian study.[13] In general, however, neuritis was not found to be more severe in HIV-positive cases.[14] A few case reports of ENL in coinfected patients have been published. Co-infected patients with reactions appear to need very long courses of steroid treatment.[13,14] Patients with HIV are also at risk of developing peripheral nerve damage including generalized peripheral neuropathy and mono-neuritis multiplex through several mechanisms, namely, treatment with antiretrovirals and

London School of Hygiene and Tropical Medicine, Keppel Street, WC1E 7HT London, UK
* Corresponding author.
E-mail address: Diana.Lockwood@lshtm.ac.uk

Dermatol Clin 29 (2011) 125–128
doi:10.1016/j.det.2010.08.016
0733-8635/11/$ – see front matter © 2011 Published by Elsevier Inc.

derm.theclinics.com

HIV infection per se. In analogy to the situation for tuberculosis in HIV coinfected individuals, it was assumed that HIV coinfection would worsen nerve damage in leprosy patients. There are a few early studies reporting no increase in nerve damage in coinfected patients.[12–14] A well controlled study of peripheral nerve function in coinfected patients would be useful. **Table 1** summarizes the expected versus actual impact of HIV-1 on coinfected patients.

IMMUNOLOGY OF HIV AND LEPROSY COINFECTION

Patients with tuberculoid leprosy have good cell-mediated immune response to M leprae, resulting in a few skin lesions, which histologically have well organized lymphocyte (CD68+, CD3+, CD8+, CD4+)-rich granulomas with predominantly CD4 T cells. In contrast, patients with LL have a strong humoral response but poor or absent cell-medicated immunity, resulting in uncontrolled growth of bacilli and disseminated skin lesions. Histologic examination of biopsies from their lesions reveals that the granulomas are comprised of macrophages and small numbers of CD8 T cells.[10]

HIV affects cell-mediated immunity, and it was initially expected that, just as in M. tuberculosis infection, the decrease in CD4 cells would result in decreased capacity for mycobacterial containment and thus an increase in disseminated disease. But studies have shown that HIV coinfected patients with low CD4 count had borderline tuberculoid lesions with well formed granuloma and normal CD4 cells numbers. In contrast, coinfected patients with LL lesions showed loose infiltrates comprised of macrophages and a small number of almost exclusively CD8 lymphocytes.[15,16] Carvalho and colleagues[16] found that the coinfected group exhibits lower CD4 to CD8 ratios, higher levels of CD8+ activation, increased Vδ1 to Vδ2 T cell ratios and decreased percentages of plasmacytoid dendritic cells as compared with HIV-1 mono-infected patients. The exact immunopathological mechanism underlying the possible increase in frequency of leprosy reactions is not clear. Dysregu-lation of the immune system and the heightened state of immune activation in HIV infection may be responsible. In addition, delayed clearance of M.leprae antigen caused by impaired phagocytic function of macrophages also has been implicated.

EFFECT OF ANTIRETROVIRAL THERAPY ON HIV AND LEPROSY COINFECTION

Since the introduction of highly active antiretroviral therapy (HAART) in the management of HIV, especially in regions endemic for leprosy, co-infected patients are also developing tuberculoid leprosy with active lesions, and ulceration of lesions is seen in leprosy type 1 reactions. Leprosy is being increasingly reported as part of the immune recon-stitution inflammatory syndrome (IRIS).

IRIS is a paradoxic deterioration in clinical status after starting HAART, a deterioration that is attribut-able to the recovery or reactivation of someone's immune response to a latent or subclinical process. The HAART regimes currently used increase production and redistribution of CD4+ cells and improve pathogen-specific immunity, both to HIV and other pathogens. While improved immunity to HIV is the required effect from HAART, improved immunity to other opportunistic pathogens or development of autoimmunity can result in IRIS. The prevalence of IRIS in cohort studies of HIV-positive patients ranges from 3% to more than 50%, varying greatly with the acquired immunode-ficiency syndrome (AIDS)- defining illness affecting the patient at the start of HAART therapy.[17] Risk factors for the development of IRIS include advanced HIV disease with a CD4+ T cell count

Table 1
Summary of impact of human immunodeficiency virus-1 on leprosy: expected versus actual

		Theory	In Practice
Epidemiologic	Incidence	Increase in leprosy	No change
Clinical	Tuberculoid leprosy	Decreased	Increased
	Treatment response	Worsened	No change
	Type-1 reactional states	Fewer	Increased
	Neuritis	Worsened	?
	Novel findings	Presentation as immune reconstitution inflammatory syndrome	
Histopathological	Granuloma formation	Decreased	No change
	Bacterial index	Increased	No change

under 50 cells/mm, unrecognized opportunistic infection or high microbial burden, and the number and presence of prior opportunistic infections. HAART triggers overt clinical manifestations of coinfection with tuberculosis, cytomegalovirus, herpes zoster, C and B hepatitis virus, and now leprosy.

Since 2003, 23 reports of patients developing leprosy as IRIS have been published.[2,3,15-19] Most patients had borderline leprosy, and type 1 reactions frequently occurred. Ulceration, a highly unusual feature in leprosy lesions, was observed in six patients, and four patients also developed neuritis. It may be that the high proportion of borderline tuberculoid leprosy cases among the HIV-infected patients on HAART could shed light on the questions related to the kinetics of M leprae infection and development of disease. Borderline tuberculoid leprosy manifests 2 to 5 years after infection, at which time specific cell-mediated immunity is strong enough to cause tissue damage as well as kill or at least control mycobacterial growth. On the other hand, lepromatous (BL and LL) forms appear in patients after longer periods of incubation (5 to 10 years), during which time a large number of bacilli have accumulated in the tissue due to progressive reduction of CMI. Although HIV patients are typically more aware of their health status and would easily detect small lesions, the high frequency of borderline tuberculoid patients and reactions among HIV-infected individuals and the low bacillary load among the co-infected MB patients strongly suggest an earlier-than-usual detection of the disease in immune-reconstituted patients.

To facilitate the recognition and classification of leprosy-associated IRIS, the following case definition has been suggested[20]:

> Leprosy or leprosy reaction presenting within 6 months of starting HAART
> Advanced HIV infection
> Low CD4+ count before starting HAART
> CD4+ count increasing after HAART has been started.

Subdividing leprosy-associated IRIS into groups according to data on timing and clinical presentation may help toward defining the causes and mechanisms of this phenomenon. Deps and Lockwood[21] recently proposed such a subdivision, attempting to separate unmasking episodes from those of overlap of immune restoration.

There are several possible mechanisms for the pathogenesis of leprosy IRIS. Leprosy has a long incubation period, and HAART may provide the immunologic trigger for normal disease. Another explanation is that leprosy-associated IRIS is similar to a type 1 reaction. Whatever the underlying mechanisms, it is likely that leprosy-associated IRIS will be increasingly reported, especially as access to HAART becomes more widely available. There are also several case reports of patients being diagnosed with leprosy more than 6 months after the initiation of HAART. Although these patients can present with any kind of leprosy, including histoid leprosy,[22] the time lag of greater than 6 months since the initiation of HAART excludes the diagnosis of IRIS.

SUMMARY

From the available data so far, one can conclude that treatment of leprosy patients with concurrent HIV infection does not differ from that of a seronegative leprosy patient: standard WHO-MDT, in conjunction with HAART if the CD4 count is low. Treatment of reactions can be managed with corticosteroids or thalidomide as appropriate.

There are currently no good prospective clinical data on the clinical features of leprosy in HIV-infected patients, particularly the evolution of their skin lesions and progression of nerve damage and response to MDT. The inclusion of HIV testing in sentinel studies of patients relapsing after multidrug therapy treatment would give some indication as to whether HIV infection is an important cofactor in relapse. Response to treatment for neuritis and reaction in coinfected patients needs to be studied carefully in prospective studies.

The influence of HIV infection on cell-mediated immune responses to M leprae in the HIV-infected patient needs exploration, especially within the skin. The recognition of leprosy presenting as IRIS warrants immunologic studies, using, for example, immunohistochemistry to delineate cellular phenotypes within the granuloma and mRNA and protein production to assess cytokine expression.

Leprosy and HIV coinfection is an evolving situation with ongoing discoveries and further research needs.

REFERENCES

1. Ustianowski AP, Lawn SD, Lockwood DN. Interactions between HIV infection and leprosy: a paradox. Lancet Infect Dis 2006;6(6):350–60.
2. Lawn SD, Wood C, Lockwood DN. Borderline tuberculoid leprosy: an immune reconstitution phenomenon in a human immunodeficiency virus-infected person. Clin Infect Dis 2003;36(1):e5–6.

3. Couppie P, Abel S, Voinchet H, et al. Immune reconstitution inflammatory syndrome associated with HIV and leprosy. Arch Dermatol 2004;140(8):997–1000.
4. Lucas S. Human immunodeficiency virus and leprosy. Lepr Rev 1993;64:97–103.
5. Leonard G, Sangare A, Verdier M, et al. Prevalence of HIV infection among patients with leprosy in African countries and Yemen. J Acquir Immune Defic Syndr 1990;3:1109–13.
6. Ponnighaus JM, Mwanjasi LJ, Fine PE, et al. Is HIV infection risk factor for leprosy? Int J Lepr 1991;59: 221–8.
7. Borgdorff MW, van der Broek J, Chum HJ, et al. HIV-1 infection as a risk factor for leprosy; a case control study in Tanzania. Int J Lepr Other Mycobact Dis 1993;61:556–62.
8. Orege PA, Fine PE, Lucas SB, et al. A case control study on human immunodeficiency virus-1 (HIV-1) infection as a risk for tuberculosis and leprosy in western Kenya. Tuber Lung Dis 1993;74:3777–81.
9. Sarno EN, Illarramendi X, Nery JA, et al. HIV-M. leprae interaction: can HAART modify the course of leprosy? Public Health Rep 2008;123:206–12.
10. Pereira GAS, Stefani MMA, Araújo Filho JA, et al. Human immunodeficiency virus type 1 (HIV-1) and Mycobacterium leprae coinfection: HIV-1 subtypes and clinical, immunologic and histopathologic profiles in a Brazilian cohort. Am J Trop Med Hyg 2004;71(5):679–84.
11. Rath N, Kar HK. Leprosy in HIV infection: a study of three cases. Indian J Lepr 2003;75:355–9.
12. Birwe R, Kawuma HJ. Type 1 reactions in leprosy, neuritis and steroid therapy: the impact of the human immunodeficiancy virus. Trans R Soc Trop Med Hyg 1994;88:315–6.
13. Talhari C, Mira MT, Massone C, et al. Leprosy and HIV: a clinical, pathological, immunological and therapeutic study of a cohort from a Brazilian referral centre and infectious diseases. J Infect Dis 2010; 202:345–54.
14. Lockwood DN, Lambert S. HIV and leprosy: where are we at? Lepr Rev 2010;81:167–75.
15. Sampaio EP, Caneshi JRT, Nery JA, et al. Cellular immune response to Mycobacterium leprae infection in human immunodeficiency virus-infected individuals. Infect Immun 1995;63:1848–54.
16. Carvalho KL, Maeda S, Marti L, et al. Immune cellular parameters of leprosy and human immunodeficiency virus-1 c-infected subjects. Immunology 2008;124:206–14.
17. Muller M, Wandel S, Colebunders R, et al. Immune reconstitution inflammatory syndrome in patients starting antiretroviral therapy for HIV infection: a systematic review and meta-analysis. Lancet Infect Dis 2010;10:251–61.
18. Lawn SD, Lockwood DN. Leprosy after starting antiretroviral treatment. BMJ 2007;334(7587):217–8.
19. Vinay K, Smita J, Nikhil G, et al. Human Immunodeficiency virus and leprosy coinfection in Pune, India. J Clin Microbiol 2009;47(9):2998–9.
20. Deps PD, Lockwood DN. Leprosy occurring as immune reconstitution syndrome. Trans R Soc Trop Med Hyg 2008;102(10):966–8.
21. Deps PD, Lockwood DN. Leprosy presenting as immune reconstitution inflammatory syndrome: proposed definitions and classification. Lepr Rev 2010;81:59–68.
22. Bumb RA, Ghiya BC, et al. Histoid leprosy in a patient of acquired immune-deficiency syndrome taking HAART. Lepr Rev 2010.

Index

Dermatol Clin 29 (2011) 129–134
doi:10.1016/S0733-8635(10)00191-9

derm.theclinics.com